Pancreatic Cancer - Updates in Pathogenesis, Diagnosis and Therapies

Edited by Emad Hamdy Gad

Published in London, United Kingdom

Pancreatic Cancer - Updates in Pathogenesis, Diagnosis and Therapies
http://dx.doi.org/10.5772/intechopen.104151
Edited by Emad Hamdy Gad

Contributors
Kmira Zahra, Wided Cherif, Haifa Regaieg, Monia Zaier, Yosra Ben Youssef, Abderrahim Khelif, Naila Fathallah, Azize Saroglu, Alexander Julianov, Kai Sun, Nikitha Vobugari, Michele Molinari, Hao Liu, Christof Kaltenmeier, Maen A. Abdelrahim, Mohamed Badheeb, Abdullah Esmail, Emad Hamdy Gad

First published in London, United Kingdom, 2023 by IntechOpen
IntechOpen is the global imprint of INTECHOPEN LIMITED, registered in England and Wales, registration number: 11086078, 5 Princes Gate Court, London, SW7 2QJ, United Kingdom

British Library Cataloguing-in-Publication Data
A catalogue record for this book is available from the British Library

Additional hard and PDF copies can be obtained from orders@intechopen.com

Pancreatic Cancer - Updates in Pathogenesis, Diagnosis and Therapies
Edited by Emad Hamdy Gad
p. cm.
Print ISBN 978-1-80355-921-6
Online ISBN 978-1-80355-922-3
eBook (PDF) ISBN 978-1-80355-923-0

For EU product safety concerns:
IN TECH d.o.o., Prolaz Marije Krucifikse Kozulić 3, 51000 Rijeka, Croatia,
info@intechopen.com or visit our website at intechopen.com.

Meet the editor

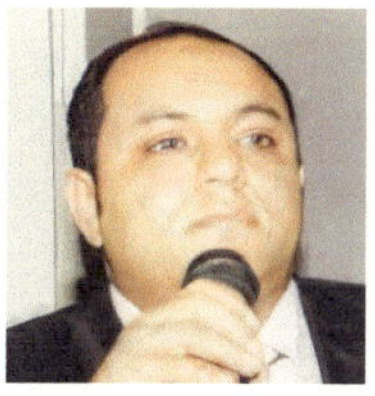

Dr. Emad Hamdy Gad works as a professor of hepatobiliary surgery in the Transplantation, Hepatobiliary and Pancreatic Surgery Department, National Liver Institute, Menoufia University, Menoufia, Egypt. He was involved in the management of liver transplantation patients and shared in over (400) Living-related liver transplantation (LRLT), pediatrics and adults at the National Liver Institute, University of Menoufia. Menoufia, Egypt. He worked as a consultant general, hepatopancreatobiliary and laparoscopic surgery in King Khaled Hospital (General surgery and trauma hospital) in Hail in KSA for 6 months (Locum) from 2/ 2015 to 8/2015. He worked as a consultant in general surgery at Alnile Hospital, Gherghada, Egypt from 3/2016 until 8/2016. He worked as a consultant general and hepatobiliary surgeon at King Faisal Hospital, Taif, KSA from 8/2016 until 8/2019. He is one of the editorial board members of different international journals like *Advances in Medical Oncology Research* (AMOR) journal, *Journal of Oncology Research and Therapy* (ISSN 2574-710X), *Henry Journal of Cellular and Molecular Oncology, Austin Hepatology journal*, etc. He is a reviewer in some Q1 journals like the *World Journal of Gastroenterology, World Journal of Surgery*, etc. He is the author of numerous international papers, which have had a significant influence in the academic community. Notably, his research profile on RCA (Reference Citation Analysis) can be accessed at this link(https://referencecitationanalysis.com/00001195) where he has garnered a total of 346 citations in Crossref. On ResearchGate (RG), he boasts an Research Interest Score of 679.9, along with 656 citations and an h-index of 9. His Google Scholar h-index stands at 9, with 303 citations. Additionally, his Scopus h-index is 7, supported by 155 citations. For more information, you can visit his ORCID profile at this link(https://orcid.org/0000-0003-1993-6899).

Contents

Preface

Despite the progress in pancreatic cancer (PC) chemo/radiotherapies, immunotherapies, and novel targeted therapies, as well as the improvement in its perioperative management policies, it is still a deadly and challenging catastrophic tumor with a high mortality rate, even after radical resection. It has a notable bad prognosis in comparison to other malignant tumors due to its high degree of malignancy, gradual onset, typical symptoms defect, delayed discovery, difficult anatomical location, early neural and vascular invasions, early micro-metastatic spread, tumor heterogeneities, unique desmoplastic stroma and tumor microenvironment (TME), high rate of chemo/radiotherapy resistance, lower rate of curative resection, and its tendency to recur after resection. Globally, PC is the seventh leading cause of cancer-related mortality.

The most common cancer of the pancreas is pancreatic duct adenocarcinoma (PDAC), which accounts for more than 90% of all cancers. Both the occurrence and progression of PDAC come from changes in some genes (i.e., KRAS oncogene mutational activation, inactivation of tumor suppressor genes (CDKN2A, TP53 and SMAD4), and/or mutations in other genes involved in the cell cycle and apoptosis). Other risk factors include lifestyle factors (i.e., tobacco use, alcohol, obesity, diabetes, chronic pancreatitis, etc.) as well as some precancerous lesions (i.e., pancreatic intraepithelial neoplasia (PanIN), intra-ductal papillary mucinous neoplasm (IPMN), mucinous cystic neoplasms (MCN), etc.)

Besides PDAC, there are other pathological types of pancreatic cancers, such as acinar cell carcinoma, small cell carcinoma, cystadenocarcinoma, pancreatoblastoma, pancreatic neuroendocrine tumor (PNET), and others.

PC can be diagnosed clinically (i.e., jaundice, dark urine, clay stool, abdominal pain, unexplained weight loss, etc.), by laboratory measures (i.e., carbohydrate antigen (CA19-9), etc.), by imaging (endoscopic ultrasonography (EUS), abdominal magnetic resonance imaging (MRI) and/or multi-detector computed tomography (MDCT) with pancreatic protocols, etc.), and by pathological detection (pancreatic biopsy).

Understanding tumor pathogenesis at the detailed genetic/epigenetic/metabolic/molecular levels as well as studying the tumor risk factors and its known precancerous lesions is required for successful treatment. In addition, early diagnosis and treatment by a multidisciplinary team of surgeons, gastroenterologists/interventional upper endoscopists, medical/radiation oncologists, diagnostic/intervention radiologists, and pathologists at high-volume centers is important for better outcomes. Moreover, surgical resection with a negative margin (R0) is the only cure for PC.

According to tumor stage; resectable cancers are treated by surgical resection followed by adjuvant therapy. On the other hand; borderline resectable tumors are treated by neoadjuvant therapy followed by surgical resection. However, for patients with locally advanced or distant metastatic pancreatic cancers, FOLFIRINOX (fluorouracil (5-FU), leucovorin, irinotecan and oxaliplatin) and/or gemcitabine (a nucleotide analogue) plus albumin-bound paclitaxel (nab-paclitaxel) have been approved for use with high success. Lastly, future targeted therapies depending upon molecular pathways, tumor gene mutations, and modulation of the tumor microenvironment (TME) are currently being studied in clinical trials.

This book discusses PC, focusing on its pathogenesis, risk factors, pathology, diagnosis, and treatment. It is organized into four sections. The first section includes an introductory chapter about PC prevention, screening, and detection. The second section examines the pathogenesis and risk factors of PC. The third section discusses cancer pathogenesis, pathology, and management. Finally, the fourth section presents pancreatitis in children.

Overall, the book provides updated knowledge about the pathogenesis, prevention, screening, detection, and treatment of this catastrophic cancer.

Emad Hamdy Gad, MBChB, MD, MSc, Doctor, Professor, Surgeon
Professor of Hepatobiliary Surgery,
National Liver Institute,
Menoufia University,
Menoufia, Egypt

Section 1

Introduction

Chapter 1

Introductory Chapter: Pancreatic Cancer – How to Prevent, Screen, and Detect?

Emad Hamdy Gad

1. Introduction

Pancreatic cancer is a very rapidly invasive/metastatic tumor having a poor response to the standard therapies. It has a very poor prognosis; moreover, pancreatic ductal adenocarcinoma (PDAC), the most common and aggressive type of pancreatic cancer (PC), has the lowest 5-year survival rate among all known cancers globally. This poor prognosis comes from cancer late presentation due to non-specific symptoms (i.e., weight loss, abdominal pain, nausea, fatigue) leading to its discovery at late advanced/metastatic stages (i.e., around 80% of patients have distant metastases when diagnosed) precluding its effective curative surgical resection resulting in its catastrophic bad outcome [1]. So, it is fundamental to have new tools for prevention, screening, and proper early detection of this challenging cancer for improving its outcome.

PC is classified pathologically into adenocarcinomas (>90%), cystadenocarcinomas, mucinous tumors, and lastly, the neuroendocrine tumors (NET) that have the best prognosis [1]. It can be diagnosed clinically (i.e., jaundice, dark urine, clay stool, abdominal pain, unexplained weight loss), by laboratory measures (i.e., carbohydrate antigen (CA19–9)), imaging (endoscopic ultrasonography (EUS), abdominal magnetic resonance imaging (MRI), and/or multi-detector computed tomography (MDCT) with pancreatic protocols), and pathological detection (pancreatic biopsy) [2].

Our book discusses some recent issues related to pancreatic cancer with stress on its pathogenesis, risk factors, pathology, diagnosis, and treatment, where we sorted it into four sectors; the first sector includes an introductory chapter about pancreatic cancer prevention, screening, and detection, the second sector contains pathogenesis and risk factors of cancer, while the third sector includes cancer pathogenesis, pathology, and management, and finally, the fourth sector is about miscellaneous pancreatic topics.

This introductory chapter gives some recent hints about the updated data on the prevention, screening, and detection of this catastrophic cancer.

2. Prevention

PC can be prevented by lifestyle modification and by acting on and modulating its modifiable risk factors (i.e., smoking, obesity, physical inactivity, diabetes

IntechOpen

mellitus (DM), alcohol abuse) [3, 4]; moreover, it can be prevented by high vegetables/fruits/nuts/whole grain diets as well as by low fat/calory diets [5]. Regarding chemoprevention of PC, metformin is a good example as it acts on different organs/tissues in diabetic and/or obese patients (i.e., liver, gut, skeletal muscle, fat) leading to decreased levels of blood glucose, insulin and insulin growth factor (IGF), reduced food intake, weight loss, as well as changes in the gut microbiome (microbiota having a role in PC pathogenesis), as a sequence, leading to prevention of PDAC development. Furthermore, phytochemicals like curcumin may have a role in its prevention [6].

3. Screening and surveillance

Selective screening of the non-symptomatic persons at high risk for cancer pancreas is required for early discovery of the high-grade precancerous lesions (e.g., pancreatic intraepithelial neoplasia (PanIN-3) or cystic lesions (intra-ductal papillary mucinous neoplasm (IPMN)/mucinous cystic neoplasm (MCN) with high-grade dysplasia) or the early stage cancer that can be resected with a high survival rate. Moreover, screening is associated with better cures/survivals and lower unnecessary/overtreatments if performed using better diagnostic tools, and through multidisciplinary teams qualified in pancreatic surgery, radiology, endoscopy, pathology, as well as genetics. Also, it has a positive effect on personal quality of life (QOL), cancer worry, and psychological distress [2, 7, 8].

The high-risk PC patients that should undergo screening are first-degree relatives (FDRs) of familial pancreatic cancer(FPC)patients, patients with Peutz-Jeghers syndrome (PJS) or Familial atypical multiple-mole melanoma syndrome (FAMMM) irrespective of family history of PC, carriers of breast cancer susceptibility (BRCA2, BRCA1), partner and localizer of BRCA2(PALB2), and ataxia telangiectasia mutated (ATM) gene mutation with ≥1 affected FDR, carriers of mismatch repair(MMR) gene mutation with ≥1 affected FDR, as well as incidentally discovered pancreatic cystic lesions [2, 7, 8].

The screening should start at 35–40 years of age in PJS and FAMMM cases, at 45 years in other detected mutations of hereditary pancreatic cancer (HPC) syndromes(i.e., mutations of BRCA2, BRCA1, PALB2, ATM genes) and at 50 years of age or 10 years younger than the earliest age of PC in FPC cases. Moreover, it should be performed twice a year. EUS ± fine needle aspiration cytology/biopsy (FNAC/B) and MRI/magnetic resonance cholangiopancreatography (MRCP) are the recently advised initial screening tools. However, other non-common screening tools are MDCT, positron emission tomography (PET)/CT, and endoscopic retrograde cholangiopancreatography (ERCP) ± brush cytology. Nevertheless, the previous screening tools have remarkable false-positive or false-negative results leading to unnecessary or delayed management, respectively [2, 4, 7].

In addition to the previously mentioned screening tools, there are other promising tools under investigation (e.g., contrast-enhanced EUS, EUS elastography (tissue stiffness measurement), CA19–9 + thrombospondin-2(multifunctional family of glycoproteins that regulates tumor migration and invasion), circulating tumor DNA, radiomics (extraction of information from certain medical images by advanced feature analysis)) [9].

4. Diagnosis, staging, and early detection of PC

The earlier the diagnosis of PC, the more possibility of well-differentiated, nodal free, smaller tumors with non-vascular non-neural invasions leading to better outcomes; so, multiple recent efforts have been made in different directions for getting early diagnostic PC tools; they include serological tests, genetic mutation marker analysis, DNA/RNA/protein markers, imaging (EUS/CT/MRI/ERCP) tools, diagnostic laparoscopy, as well as histopathological tools [10].

Clinically and according to PC location, it can be manifested by abdominal pain, back pain, shoulder pain, nausea, vomiting, weight loss, bloating, dyspepsia, dysphagia, bowel habit changes, pruritus, jaundice, steatorrhea, lethargy, new-onset diabetes, and depression. However, cancer patients may be asymptomatic and patients with pancreatic body/tail cancers may have late presentation [1, 11].

Serologically, a complete blood count and complete metabolic panel (i.e., liver function tests (LFT), coagulation profile, serum markers, pancreatic juice markers) are required for serological detection of PC.

CA19-9 is a carbohydrate antigen widely used as a serum biomarker for PC and it is still the current standard serum tumor marker; however, it has some limitations (i.e., low sensitivity and specificity, expressed only in individuals with Lewis a+/b- or Lewis a+/b + genotypes, elevated also in some non-cancerous conditions as pancreatitis and in many non-pancreatic malignancies, poor in the screening of symptomatic patients). Nevertheless, its combination with other serum markers like cell migration-inducing protein (CEMIP), CA125, carcinoembryonic antigen (CEA), and K-RAS gene mutation markers may improve its accuracy in diagnosing PC [12, 13].

CA-242 is a sialylated carbohydrate antigen elevated in some tumors like pancreatic cancers and its combination with CA19–9 leads to higher sensitivities and specificities in diagnosing PC. Similarly, other serum markers like hematopoietic growth factors (HGFs), alcohol dehydrogenase (ADH), tissue polypeptide-specific antigen (TPS), pancreatic cancer-specific antigen (PAA), D-dimer (DD), fibrinogen (FIB), and beta 2-microglobulin (beta 2-MG) may be elevated in PC. In addition to the previous markers, pancreatic juice CEA elevation can detect pancreatic cancer with acceptable accuracy [11, 12, 14].

Recently, new agents like DNA biomarkers (i.e., mutant TP53/SMAD4(tumor suppressor genes)) in pancreatic juice, and circulating-tumor DNA (cell-free DNA(cfDNA)) in serum), RNA biomarkers(e.g., microRNAs (miRNAs); non-coding RNA molecules regulating gene expression at mRNA levels either by their degradation or by translational inhibition), protein markers (osteopontin (OPN)), circulating tumor cells, exosomes (extracellular vesicle containing cellular constituents such as DNA, RNA, protein, and lipids secreted by all cell types into the circulation to transport biological components to other cells regulating intercellular communication), as well as microbiota (living microorganisms that normally inhabit human bodies mainly gastrointestinal tracts (GITs)) have been developed for the early detection of PC; however, their sensitivities and specificities remain under investigations [2].

Cell-free DNAs (cfDNAs) are double-stranded DNA molecules circulating in the blood. They are released during normal cellular metabolism, apoptosis, or necrosis. PC patients have a significant level of cfDNA in their blood. The detection of cfDNA tumor-specific mutations (e.g., KRAS mutation) and/or epigenetic alteration by methods such as digital PCR, peptide-nucleic acid clamp PCR, and panel sequencing in the serum of PC patients is a promising diagnostic tool [15].

Recent rapid diagnostic technologies (e.g., *in situ* hybridization, oligonucleotide microarrays, northern blotting with radiolabelled probes, deep/parallel sequencing, TaqMan assays (qPCR-based detection of miRNAs)) have been used to perform miRNA expression profiling for early detection of PC through samples taken from PC tissues, serum/plasma, and pancreatic juice with high accuracy rate. Moreover, the increased serum levels of certain miRNAs like miR-16 and miR-196a in combination with elevated serum CA19-9 have higher accuracy in detecting early PC. On the other hand; some other miRNAs like miR-1290 have a better diagnostic accuracy of early PC than CA19-9 [16, 17].

Osteopontin (OPN) is an extracellular matrix protein (ECM) having a role in cell adhesion, migration, and apoptosis. It is upregulated in PC and linked to cancer invasiveness and metastasis. Its serum level is elevated in PC with acceptable accuracy [15].

Circulating tumor cells (CTCs) are tumor cells that originated from a primary tumor into circulation. They are involved in the distant metastatic character of the tumor. They can be used as potential serum biomarkers for PDAC [18].

Exosomes are perfect promising future PC diagnostic tool due to the following: 1—They are produced frequently by PC cells, 2—they can be non-invasively collected from different body fluids, 3—they can be re-collected over time for monitoring, 4—they are stable, and their contents of proteins and nucleic acids are protected from destruction by external nucleases and proteases, and 5—they can be detected easily by sensitive modern technologies. The exosomal glypican-1 (GPC1), zinc transporter protein (ZIP4), miR-196a, miR-1246, mutant KRAS, and Mutant TP53 are examples of those exosomal diagnostic biomarkers [19, 20].

The microbiota that normally inhabits human mouth and colon undergo changes in PDAC; analysis of those microbiotal changes (dysbiosis) as well as their metabolites through salivary and fecal samples can be used as a non-invasive tools for early detection of PDAC [21].

Abdominal ultrasound (US) can be a tool for the diagnosis of PC patients despite the difficulty due to the retroperitoneal pancreatic location. Being cost-effective and non-invasive, US can be used as a screening method for early detection of pancreatic cancer where the tumor appears as a hypoechoic mass. Moreover, US-guided fine needle aspiration cytology/biopsy (FNAC/B) and DNA analysis of the lesion can also be performed [11].

EUS is more accurate in detecting pancreatic tumor shape, morphology, internal echo, LNs, vascular relations and bile duct changes. Along with MDCT, EUS is considered excellent tool in preoperative staging of PC. Moreover, EUS-guided FNAC/B can be done safely, effectively, and easily with higher accuracy in distinguishing benign from malignant lesions. Furthermore, novel techniques of EUS-FNAC/B, such as fanning and slow-pull techniques with or without liquid-based cytology, have many advantages (i.e., higher detection accuracy, getting more material for histological diagnosis, better detection of KRAS mutation, microRNA profiling) [11, 14, 22].

Accurate tumor diagnosis and staging can be done through angiographic MDCT with pancreatic protocol with advanced volumetric techniques to detect small lesions, and to reach the relationship between the tumor and the neighboring vessels (i.e., celiac axis and superior mesenteric vessels) [11, 14]. Moreover, in MDCT pancreatic protocol, the reconstructed slice thickness should be 3 mm without gap with 3D volumetric images for vascular assessment. It is done in dual phase pattern: the pancreatic parenchymal phase (40 to 50 sec) and the portal venous phase (65 to 70 sec). Maximal pancreatic parenchyma enhancement and adequate arterial opacification are obtained in the first phase, while porto-mesentric venous and liver opacifications are achieved in the other phase [23].

PET is accurate in localizing primary and metastatic lesions depending upon increased FDG uptake by tumor in comparison with normal tissue. If combined with CT (PET/CT), the diagnostic accuracy increases. It is recommended in screening of high-risk patients of pancreatic cancer for detecting extra pancreatic metastases after the standard screening tools [11, 14].

MRI either gadolinium-enhanced MRI or diffusion-weighted imaging (DWI)-MRI are similar to helical CT regarding sensitivities and specificities, and in determining tumor resectability; moreover, the non-invasive MRCP is an excellent delineator of the pancreatic and biliary ducts [11, 14, 22]. In addition to the previous MRI tools, PET-MRI is a newer technique providing more information regarding cancer spread to the main pancreatic duct, collateral veins, superior mesenteric artery, celiac artery, and the liver [24].

ERCP-guided brushing cytology and aspiration cytology are good diagnostic tools of PC; furthermore, ERCP-probe-based confocal laser endomicroscopy and ERCP-guided serial pancreatic juice aspiration cytologic examination (SPACE) have high sensitivities in detecting malignant pancreaticobiliary strictures and pancreatic carcinoma *in situ* (PCIS), respectively [22, 25].

Staging laparoscopy may be needed through a case-by-case basis, especially in patients with a high suspicious of occult metastatic disease (i.e., body/tail tumors, large tumors (>3 cm), suspected LN involvement in the image, and a very high CA 19–9 [24]).

Lastly, the pathological diagnosis is required for non-operative non-resectable cases to draw a suitable treatment plan of chemo/radio/immune therapies. In addition, it may be required preoperatively to give the proper neo-adjuvant therapies. The pathological samples may be US, EUS, CT, or laparoscopic guided biopsies (FNAC/B, true cut biopsy, etc.) taken from the primary lesion, the regional/metastatic LNs, the metastatic lesion or from ascites [13, 26].

Finally, I think our book will give the readers important knowledge about pancreatic cancer.

Author details

Emad Hamdy Gad
Hepatobiliary and Liver Transplantation Surgery Department, National Liver Institute, Menoufia University, Menoufia, Egypt

*Address all correspondence to: emadgadsalemaa@yahoo.com

References

[1] Nattress CB, Halldén G. Advances in oncolytic adenovirus therapy for pancreatic cancer. Cancer Letters. 2018;**434**:56-69. DOI: 10.1016/j.canlet.2018.07.006

[2] Wood LD, Canto MI, Jaffee EM, Simeone DM. Pancreatic cancer: Pathogenesis, screening, diagnosis, and treatment. Gastroenterology. 2022;**163**(2):386-402.e1. DOI: 10.1053/j.gastro.2022.03.056

[3] Bartolini I, Nannini G, Risaliti M, Matarazzo F, Moraldi L, Ringressi MN, et al. Impact of microbiota-immunity axis in pancreatic cancer management. World Journal of Gastroenterology. 2022;**28**(32):4527-4539. DOI: 10.3748/wjg.v28.i32.4527

[4] Olakowski M, Bułdak Ł. Current status of inherited pancreatic cancer. Hered Cancer Clinical Practise. 2022;**20**(1):26. DOI: 10.1186/s13053-022-00224-2

[5] Mohammed A, Janakiram NB, Pant S, Rao CV. Molecular targeted intervention for pancreatic cancer. Cancers (Basel). 2015;7(3):1499-1542. DOI: 10.3390/cancers7030850

[6] Eibl G, Rozengurt E. Metformin: Review of epidemiology and mechanisms of action in pancreatic cancer. Cancer Metastasis Reviews. 2021;**40**(3):865-878. DOI: 10.1007/s10555-021-09977-z

[7] Chen F, Roberts NJ, Klein AP. Inherited pancreatic cancer. China Clinical Oncology. 2017;**6**(6):58. DOI: 10.21037/cco.2017.12.04

[8] Torphy RJ, Fujiwara Y, Schulick RD. Pancreatic cancer treatment: Better, but a long way to go. Surgery Today. 2020;**50**(10):1117-1125. DOI: 10.1007/s00595-020-02028-0

[9] Dudley B, Brand RE. Pancreatic cancer surveillance and novel strategies for screening. Gastrointestinal Endoscopy Clinics of North America. 2022;**32**(1):13-25. DOI: 10.1016/j.giec.2021.08.008

[10] Pothuraju R, Rachagani S, Junker WM, Chaudhary S, Saraswathi V, Kaur S, et al. Pancreatic cancer associated with obesity and diabetes: An alternative approach for its targeting. Journal of Experimental & Clinical Cancer Research. 2018;**37**(1):319. DOI: 10.1186/s13046-018-0963-4

[11] Li HY, Cui ZM, Chen J, Guo XZ, Li YY. Pancreatic cancer: Diagnosis and treatments. Tumour Biology. 2015;**36**(3):1375-1384. DOI: 10.1007/s13277-015-3223-7

[12] Jelski W, Mroczko B. Biochemical diagnostics of pancreatic cancer - present and future. Clinica Chimica Acta. 2019;**498**:47-51. DOI: 10.1016/j.cca.2019.08.013

[13] Zhao Z, Liu W. Pancreatic Cancer: A review of risk factors, diagnosis, and treatment. Technology in Cancer Research & Treatment. 2020;**19**:1533. DOI: 10.1177/1533033820962117

[14] Gupta N, Yelamanchi R. Pancreatic adenocarcinoma: A review of recent paradigms and advances in epidemiology, clinical diagnosis and management. World Journal of Gastroenterology. 2021;**27**(23):3158-3181. DOI: 10.3748/wjg.v27.i23.3158

[15] Khomiak A, Brunner M, Kordes M, Lindblad S, Miksch RC, Öhlund D, et al.

Recent discoveries of diagnostic, prognostic and predictive biomarkers for pancreatic cancer. Cancers (Basel). 2020;**12**(11):3234. DOI: 10.3390/cancers12113234

[16] Rachagani S, Macha MA, Heimann N, Seshacharyulu P, Haridas D, Chugh S, et al. Clinical implications of miRNAs in the pathogenesis, diagnosis and therapy of pancreatic cancer. Advanced Drug Delivery Reviews. 2015;**81**:16-33. DOI: 10.1016/j.addr.2014.10.020

[17] Al-Shaheri FN, Alhamdani MSS, Bauer AS, Giese N, Büchler MW, Hackert T, et al. Blood biomarkers for differential diagnosis and early detection of pancreatic cancer. Cancer Treatment Reviews. 2021;**96**:102193. DOI: 10.1016/j.ctrv.2021.102193

[18] Torres C, Grippo PJ. Pancreatic cancer subtypes: A roadmap for precision medicine. Annals of Medicine. 2018;**50**(4):277-287. DOI: 10.1080/07853890.2018.1453168

[19] Qian L, Yu S, Chen Z, Meng Z, Huang S, Wang P. Functions and clinical implications of exosomes in pancreatic cancer. Biochimica Et Biophysica Acta. Reviews on Cancer. 2019;**1871**(1):75-84. DOI: 10.1016/j.bbcan.2018.11.001

[20] Zhao X, Ren Y, Lu Z. Potential diagnostic and therapeutic roles of exosomes in pancreatic cancer. Biochimica Et Biophysica Acta. Reviews on Cancer. 2020;**1874**(2):188414. DOI: 10.1016/j.bbcan.2020.188414

[21] Li JJ, Zhu M, Kashyap PC, Chia N, Tran NH, McWilliams RR, et al. The role of microbiome in pancreatic cancer. Cancer Metastasis Reviews. 2021;**40**(3):777-789. DOI: 10.1007/s10555-021-09982-2

[22] Kamisawa T, Wood LD, Itoi T, Takaori K. Pancreatic cancer. Lancet. 2016;**388**(10039):73-85. DOI: 10.1016/S0140-6736(16)00141-0

[23] Horvat N, Ryan DE, LaGratta MD, Shah PM, Do RK. Imaging for pancreatic ductal adenocarcinoma. Chinese Clinical Oncology. 2017;**6**(6):62. DOI: 10.21037/cco.2017.11.03

[24] Kommalapati A, Tella SH, Goyal G, Ma WW, Mahipal A. Contemporary Management of Localized Resectable Pancreatic Cancer. Cancers (Basel). 2018;**10**(1):24. DOI: 10.3390/cancers10010024

[25] Kikuyama M, Kamisawa T, Kuruma S, Chiba K, Kawaguchi S, Terada S, et al. Early diagnosis to improve the poor prognosis of pancreatic Cancer. Cancers (Basel). 2018;**10**(2):48. DOI: 10.3390/cancers10020048

[26] Milella M, Bassi C, Boggi U, Brunetti O, Cavaliere A, Crippa S, et al. Evolving pancreatic cancer treatment: From diagnosis to healthcare management. Critical Reviews in Oncology/Hematology. 2022;**169**:103571. DOI: 10.1016/j.critrevonc.2021.103571

Section 2

Pathogenesis and Risk Factors of Pancreatic Cancer

Chapter 2

Obesity and Pancreatic Cancer: Its Role in Oncogenesis

Nikitha Vobugari and Kai Sun

Abstract

Incidence rates of pancreatic cancer are increasing worldwide. The lack of screening tools, late-stage diagnosis, and resistance to chemo and radiation therapies make pancreatic cancer the fourth leading cancer-related killer. Recently, awareness has increased about obesity as a strong yet modifiable risk factor for pancreatic cancer. The prevalence of pancreatic ductal adenocarcinoma (PDAC) was significantly higher among obese patients with a body mass index of more than 35 who did not undergo bariatric surgery versus their counterparts. Global obesity rates have increased considerably over the past decades, especially since the coronavirus pandemic. There is still a lack of understanding of the mechanisms of obesity-related PDAC. Emerging evidence suggests that chronic inflammation, circulatory lipids, insulin resistance, adipokines and cytokines release, oxidative stress, and changes in the microbiome associated with obesity are linked to its initiation and progression. Obesity also potentiates driver mutations, including Kirsten Rat Sarcoma viral oncogene (Kras) in PDAC. It is also unclear why obese patients have poorer postoperative outcomes than nonobese PDAC patients highlighting the need for better mechanistic understanding. In this chapter, we aim to provide clinicians and researchers with a comprehensive overview of the carcinogenic pathogenesis of obesity in PDAC and its implications for prevention and treatment.

Keywords: obesity, pancreatic cancer, pancreas, adenocarcinoma, exocrine pancreatic cancer, pathogenesis

1. Introduction

In the United States (US), pancreatic cancer (PC) continues to have a poor prognosis due to delayed diagnosis, late-stage disease at the time of diagnosis, and limited treatment options. Since 2000, annual incidence rates have grown at a 0.6–1% in all races, both sexes, and age categories, making it the eighth most common cancer in women and the tenth most common cancer in men [1, 2]. The risk of PC increases with age. The median age of diagnosis is around 70 years old [3]. Recent incidence trends between 2000 and 2014 show a bimodal age distribution, between 20 and 29 years and >80 years [4]. The incidence is higher in males than females, with an incidence risk ratio (IRR) of 1.32; >1 for age groups >35. There may be a link between males and environmental risk factors, such as smoking and alcohol. The incidence (496,000) and deaths (466,000) in 2020 are almost equal [5]. This equal ratio has remained constant since 2010 [6]. PC accounts for 8% of all cancer-related deaths in the US and is the third leading cause after lung and colorectal cancers [7]. In the US, 5-year survival rates for all stages steadily increased from 0.9% in 1975 to 4.2% in 2011 and 10% between 2010 and 2016. Globally, the 5-year survival rates have not exceeded 10%, except for surgically resected patients; their 5-year survival rates increased from 1.5% to 17.5% [8].

The term obesity encompasses excessive fat accumulation that impairs health [9]. Indirect anthropometric measures include body mass index (BMI), waist circumference (WC), waist-hip ratio (WHR), and body fat percentage estimated skin foldness; with the BMI being the easiest and most widely used [10]. BMI ≥ 30 is considered obese. It is further classified; class 1: 30–34, class 2 35–39, and class 3 (morbid or severe obesity) ≥ 40 [11]. In the US, the age-adjusted prevalence of obesity among adults over 20 years was 41.9% between 2017 and 2020 [12]. There was a significant rise in obesity prevalence of 30.5% between 1999 and 2000, when the Centers for Disease Control and Prevention (CDC) first recognized obesity as an epidemic [9, 13]. Adult obesity prevalence spiked by 3% between March 2020 to March 2021, the first year of the coronavirus disease 2019 (COVID-19) pandemic, which coincided with higher alcohol and tobacco use, lower rates in exercise activity due to quarantine, and higher average sleep duration [14]. Obesity can foster various detrimental health problems and increase mortality from all causes, including cardiovascular diseases, and cancers. The estimated prevalence of obesity-associated cancers is 684,000 US annually, including 210,000 among men and 470,000 among women, per CDC data. The evidence of obesity-associated cancers is consistent with breast cancer in postmenopausal women, adenocarcinoma of the esophagus, colon, endometrium, gall bladder, gastric, renal cell, pancreas, thyroid, meningioma, and multiple myeloma [15, 16].

1.1 Obesity and pancreatic cancer risk

Numerous prospective, observational, and epidemiological studies have recognized obesity as an independent and modifiable risk factor for PC [17–20]. The incidence and outcomes of PC are both adversely affected by obesity [21, 22]. According to a systematic review and meta-analysis of 23 prospective studies, both general and abdominal fatness are associated with an increased PC risk with a relative risk (RR) of 1.1 [95% confidence interval (CI), 1.07–1.14], when stratified by gender and geographical location [20]. In a 12-year study by a metabolic syndrome and cancer project, obesity increased the risk of PC by 1.5 in women and no correlation was found in males [23]. In other studies, a stronger association of obesity to PC risk is found in men and further higher in smokers [22]. Confounding risk factors such as smoking and alcohol consumption in males and females may explain the contrasting findings. Higher WHR is associated with an increase in risk in women, while higher BMI is associated with an increase in risk in both men and women [17]. Incidence risk is specifically higher with a BMI ≥ 95th percentile in early adulthood and a gain of ≥10 kg/m^2 BMI in early adulthood years [24, 25]. Those with a calorie intake at the highest quartile experienced 70% higher risk than those with the lowest quartile in a case control study [26]. High BMI and underlying genetic profiles may also contribute to the elevated average PC risk among African Americans. A 20% higher risk of PC was found in African Americans than European Americans when adjusted for other risk factors [8].

PC patients with obesity in all age groups, regardless of disease stage and tumor resection status, were associated with reduced overall survival of PC with a hazard ratio 1.26 (95% CI, 0.94–1.69) [22]. The risk of early and elevated PC mortality is significantly elevated by central obesity independent of BMI during early adulthood [21, 27]. People with BMI ≥ 35 have a worse survival rate after surgery for potentially curable PDAC. According to a retrospective study, patients with a BMI >35 are 12 times more likely to have lymph node metastasis, and their chances of recurrence and death double, compared with patients with BMI <35 [28]. Considering all of the above results, it is imperative to understand the underlying pathogenesis and implement obesity-specific prevention interventions for PDAC.

2. Biologic pathogenesis

The exact biologic interlink between obesity and PC remains unclear. PDAC represents more than 90% of all PC cases [8, 29]. PDAC develops from various precursor lesions, including mucinous cystic neoplasms (MCN), intraductal papillary mucinous neoplasms (IPMN), and pancreatic intraepithelial neoplasms (PanIN). PanINs are categorized into grades 1–3 which sequentially progress into PDAC. Several in vitro and in vivo studies are ongoing to decipher the molecular foundation of obesity-associated PDAC. A number of mechanisms are proposed, including, chronic inflammation, insulin resistance, circulatory lipids, adipokine and cytokine release, hormonal factors such as elevation of insulin-like growth factor 1 (IGF-1) and sex hormones, oxidative stress, changes in intestinal microbiome, food carcinogens, and potentiation by driver mutations. The pathogenesis is further convoluted with accumulating evidence of influence of variants in genes or genetic mutations in cell synthesis, metabolism, binding, and signaling [8, 30–32].

2.1 Obesity and potentiation of Kras activity

The activating mutations in the protooncogene Kras are the key driver mutation among 90% of the PDACs. It is the earliest genetic event in the pathogenesis noted in PanIN grade 1. In 98% of Kras mutated PDACs, missense mutations occur in glycine (G)12, G13, or glutamine71 (Q61) regions, that lead to the activation of Kras permanently [33]. In pancreatic Cre driver mice models, constitutive overexpression of active Kras G12D was identified as an important step in PanIN development and carcinogenesis [34]. Kras is found in almost all PDACs, but it is insufficient in developing PDAC. In mouse models, despite the expression of mutated Kras, mice did not readily develop into PanINs/PDACs [35]. Additional genetic, epigenetic, and tumor microenvironment alterations were required in the transformation into PDAC. The further accumulation of acquired genetic alterations in tumor suppressor genes, such as CDK2N2A, SMAD4, or TP53 contributed to the inhibition of pancreatic cell death and tumor transformation [36]. The non-genetic factors or alterations caused by other environmental factors including chronic inflammation or obesity in the tumor microenvironment are postulated to be critical steps in early steps of PanIN and progression into PDAC. Several preclinical studies have also convincingly demonstrated the accelerated transformation rates of ductal cells into PanIN among engineered obese mice [32]. In conditional KrasG12D mice model, an elevated risk of PDAC was observed among high-fat high-calorie-fed obese mice compared to normally fed non-obese mice, suggesting a synergistic effect of Kras and obesity [37]. Obesity-associated factors including insulin resistance, inflammation, and gut dysbiosis that are upstream of Kras enhance the downstream signals creating multi-loop effects [38]. Some have postulated the obesity-induced activation of signaling molecules downstream of Kras, including increased levels of phosphorylated mitogen-activated protein kinase (MEK) and extracellular signal-regulated kinases (ERK) may also be contributory [39]. Kras mutations further trigger the progression from PanIN1 to PanIN2. A positive feedback loop is created, demonstrating obesity and its tumor environment changes to be a major Kras potentiator, paving a path for prospective preventive avenues of this dismal cancer [29].

2.2 Adipokines

Adipose tissue (AT) is increasingly recognized as a dynamic hormonal and metabolically active organ that produces biologically active peptides known as adipokines. Adipocytes are capable of various internal and external cellular interactions which regulate cellular processes including food intake, insulin sensitivity, inflammation, and immune responses. Leptin and adiponectin are among the first identified and highly expressed adipokines; they are known to have opposing functions on immune cell activation [32, 40]. Other adipokines currently being evaluated include Lipocalin-2 (LCN-2), fibroblast growth factor (FGF)-21, and wingless-type mouse mammary tumor virus integration site family member 5A (Wnt5a).

Leptin is positively correlated to obesity. Higher Levels of leptin are found in women than men irrespective of BMI. Leptin plays a role in appetite control and as a pro-inflammatory modulator of pancreatic tissue. Hyperleptinemia in obesity is thought to be secondary to leptin resistance and therefore, the role of leptin in PDAC development remains controversial [41]. However, in vitro and clinical studies have demonstrated elevated serum leptin levels were higher among PDAC subjects [42]. Further studies are required to confirm its role and significance in clinical settings. Adiponectin is inversely correlated to obesity by its active role in insulin regulation, glucose and fatty acid metabolism, and overall anti-inflammatory properties. The imbalance created by adiponectin and leptin creates a pro-inflammatory pathway [40]. Several preclinical studies were consistent with adiponectin's role in pathogenesis however current evidence of adiponectin levels and PDAC is contradictory. Higher adiponectin levels correlated with lower PDAC in several prospective studies versus others showed higher levels correlated with increased risk [43, 44]. It is unclear if this is due to timing of adipokine level checking or if adipokines in pancreatic tumor environment did not correlate with serum adipokines levels, as opposed to mice studies where adipokines levels showed a positive correlation.

LCN-2 is a small extracellular protein with several biological functions including energy metabolism, inflammation, and innate immunity. Adipocytes secrete LCN-2 during metabolic stress and obesity, where LCN-2 acts as a homeostasis regulator. LCN-2 is implicated in T2DM, chronic pancreatitis, and more recently, in PDAC. Its role in both pro and anti-tumor effects has been reported. Absence of LCN-2 prevented obesity in high-fat-fed mice and decreases rate of pancreatic fibrosis, inflammation, and aberrant cell proliferation, proving its inclination toward anti-tumor activities. There is a need for more clinical studies to evaluate if LCN-2 could be a potential target in prevention of obesity and early stages of PDAC [45–47]. FGF-21 has recently come into spotlight as a regulator in glucose and lipid metabolism with the potential to treat obesity. Emerging data on its role in PDAC is underway [48]. In the presence of Kras oncogenic mutations in obese mice, FGF-21 levels were found to be significantly reduced and are implicated in the extensive inflammation, PanINs, and PDAC [49]. The intricate intracellular pathway remains unclear at this time. A pro-inflammatory adipokine, Wnt5a works in conjunction with secreted frizzled-related protein (sfrp)-5 key regulators studied in obesity. Release of Wnt5a from visceral adipose tissue (VAT) and overexpression of Wnt5a has been reported in PDAC microenvironment have shown positive correlation to downstream activity of yes-associated protein (YAP) among Kras independent aggressive squamous subtype of PDAC which operates via YAP-mediated mechanisms [50]. Further pre-clinical studies are needed to confirm such an association.

Other AT-derived cytokines include interleukin (IL)-6 and tumor necrosis factor (TNF)-alpha that is secreted by adipocytes via effect of leptin excess and macrophages in the tumor microenvironment plays a role in obesity accentuated chronic inflammatory process as well [51]. More recently, AT is studied to have effects systemically via soluble mediators released by visceral fat depots and reach pancreatic microenvironment through systemic circulation by extracellular vesicles produced by adipocytes which attach to targets on pancreatic cells [52]. It is unknown if these extracellular vesicles communicate with the precursor PanIN or PDAC cells differently from normal pancreatic cells.

Expansion and hypertrophy of AT in obesity creates an imbalance in inflammatory and anti-inflammatory cytokine release, subsequently lead to progression to PanIN and PDAC, as described in chronic inflammation section. A differential inflammatory process is well studied in visceral AT (intrabdominal fat pads, omental, mesenteric) compared to subcutaneous AT. Adipose hyperplasia is often seen in subcutaneous AT but is associated with low levels of inflammation and balanced insulin sensitivity. In contrast, hypertrophy and hyperplasia in visceral AT predominately cause the elevated pro-inflammatory response which strongly correlates with obesity-induced metabolic dysfunction and PanIN formation compared to subcutaneous AT [32, 53, 54]. The synergistic combination of elevated inflammatory response with systemic deposition of extracellular vesicles in pancreatic microenvironment is a well accepted mechanism in the pathogenesis of PDAC [54, 55]. While the differences between VAT and subcutaneous AT is well established, recent focus has driven toward intrapancreatic fat and "fatty pancreas disease" in PDAC carcinogenesis from metanalysis showing 52% pooled prevalence of intrapancreatic fat among PDAC and premalignant lesions [56]. This creates a platform for combinational effects of VAT expansion and fatty replacement of pancreas. This association remains under investigation and requires attention to guide future screening models incorporating intra-pancreatic fat measurements. A need for adequate tools to differentiate normal versus excess pancreatic fat on imaging remains a challenge.

2.3 Hormonal effects and insulin resistance

A high BMI and obesity are associated with elevated levels of insulin and C peptide levels, leading to hyperglycemia, insulin resistance, and type 2 diabetes mellitus (T2DM). All have demonstrated a role in the development of PDAC in prospective studies and meta-analysis [31, 57]. Elevated circulating and intrapancreatic insulin levels cause suppression of circulating insulin growth factor binding proteins (IGFBP)-1 and 2 and subsequently lead to higher levels of IGF-1. IGF-1 and insulin bind to IGF receptors (IGF-R) on pancreatic acinar cells and propagate cell proliferation, apoptosis, and angiogenesis [31, 58]. A crosstalk between insulin and IGF-R and G protein-coupled receptor (GPCR) signaling converges on the mechanistic target of rapamycin (mTOR) responsible for cell proliferation. Inhibitory function of metformin on insulin and IGF-R emerged its role in PDAC prevention [59, 60]. This crosstalk also stimulates YAP and transcriptional coactivator with PDZ binding motif

(TAZ) which are critical molecules in PDAC [61]. The individual levels of IGF-1, IGF-2, and IGFBP-3 did not correlate with the risk of PDAC. However, a higher IGF-1/IGFBP-3 ratio represented increased free IGF-1 which showed a significant positive trend toward elevated risk of PDAC [62]. At this time, this ratio is not routinely used as a screening tool and would need further evidence in prospective studies. In obesity, increased insulin/IGF-1 and gastrointestinal peptides that activate the GPCRs further cause increased cell proliferation. Finally, elevated levels of glucose and advanced glycation end products are known to be tumor-promoting factors and important modulators in metabolic dysfunction and carcinogenesis [63].

Stress adaptiveness of pancreatic cells is another proposed mechanism of tumorigenesis by promoting cell growth and resistance to anti-cancer therapies. Recently, stress granules (SGs) have been described, which are the intracytoplasmic condensations of proteins and mRNA driven by oxidative stress, hypoxia, endoplasmic reticulum stress, and osmotic stress. A specific pathway described where IGF1 binds to IGF-R activates S6 kinase (S6K)-1 subsequently activates serine/ arginine protein kinase (SRPK)-2 and mediates the formation of IGF-1-driven SGs among obesity-induced PDAC carcinogenesis. This pathway of SRPK-2-dependent SGs formation highlights its uniqueness and context-specific to obesity-related pathway in PDAC however needs further validation. In addition, mutant Kras upregulates the capacity of PDAC cells to form SGs, further enhancing resistance to several stimuli and chemotherapeutic agents. However, SGs are considered to cause PDAC proliferation by Kras independent pathways as well and are thought to be one of the mechanisms of PDAC resistance to Kras targeted therapy [58].

Elevated estrogen activity was observed as an initiating factor in carcinogenesis. Leptin plays a role in transcription of aromatase; a key enzyme converts androstenedione and estrone to estrogen. The data on direct activity of these steroids on androgen and estrogen receptors on pancreatic cells remains unclear in the pathogenesis of PDAC but has shown some positive cell proliferation at low levels of estrogen compared to inhibition of cell proliferation with high doses [64]. However, further studies have shown mixed expression of estrogen receptors on PDAC cells and unclear benefits with anti-estrogen therapies and prognosis [64–66].

2.4 Chronic inflammation

Obesity is a chronic subclinical pro-inflammatory state. In general, overnutrition creates an imbalance between calorie intake and energy expenditure, leading to expansion of AT. AT expansion and imbalance of adipokines leads to reduction of anti-inflammatory immune cells such as CD4+ T helper (Th) 2 cells, IL-C2s, Tregs, eosinophils, type II natural killer (NK) T cells which occur in lean state. On the other end, AT expansion leads to activation of major histocompatibility complex (MHC) II expression and myeloid cells and stimulates CD8+ Th 1 inflammatory pathway sequentially activating interferon (IFN) gamma. This immune activation causes adipocyte apoptosis and histologic changes including formation of crown-shaped clusters of engulfed macrophages which is the signature of AT inflammation [32, 67, 68]. These hypertrophied adipocytes, lymphocytes, and macrophages in the AT increase the circulatory levels of cytokines such as TNF-alpha, IL-6, leptin, and adiponectin which promote inflammation and abnormal cell growth [69]. Chronic inflammation is a key mediator of carcinogenesis noted in several cancers. Alterations in fibro-inflammatory microenvironment triggers abnormal cell proliferation, halt apoptosis, activate angiogenesis, migration, and metastasis [69]. AT can also induce insulin resistance, hyperinsulinemia, hyperglycemia, hyperlipidemia, vascular injury which are associated with oxidative stress [30].

Inflammatory cytokines and oxidative stress mainly activate the nuclear factor-kappa B (NF-kB) pathway leading to downstream activation of PanIN and PC carcinogenesis [30, 55]. Therefore, obesity-associated inflammation is a stronger risk factor for PC than chronic inflammation alone, due to this augmented interplay. Peroxisome proliferator activated receptor-gamma (PPAR-gamma), a NFkB receptor is a key regulator of pancreatic cell metabolism, cell differentiation, and anti-inflammatory role is currently being evaluated as a potential target in prevention of PDAC [30].

2.5 Gut and pancreatic microbiome

Alteration of gut microbiota is well studied in obesity-associated metabolic dysfunction and development of T2DM [70]. Obesity-associated altered gut microbiome is implicated in colorectal and hepatocellular carcinoma [71, 72]. Over the recent years, obesity-associated genetic, environmental, and nutritional factors have been implicated in the disequilibrium and crosstalks between intrapancreatic, intratumoral, and gut microbiome and its role in PDAC [55, 73–75]. Akkermansia muciniphila an intestinal symbiotic bacterium that plays a role in maintaining a functioning gut barrier and its abundance is correlated to a lower incidence of obesity and other metabolic diseases. Metformin use in preclinical studies showed reduced levels of Clostridium sensu stricto and elevated levels of Akkermansia bacteria in high-fat-fed mice, one of the possible benefits of metformin in PDAC prevention, introduced the possible underlying pathomechanism [76]. These microbiota dysbiosis causes a release of metabolites (short-chain fatty acids or lipopolysaccharides), activation of intestinal GPCRs, enabling gut permeability and translocation of bacteria/ bacterial

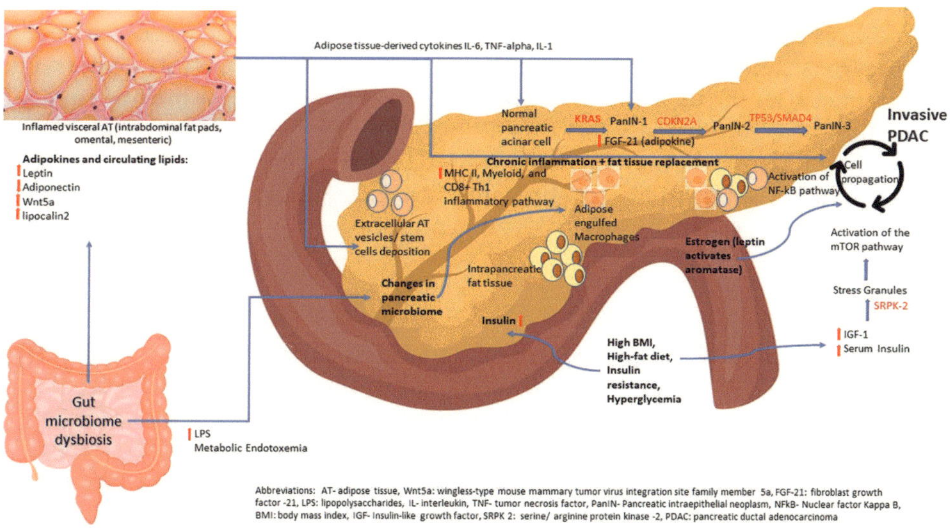

Figure 1.
Several proposed pathways of PDAC carcinogenesis. Obesity potentiates the Kras pathway via PanIN progression. Kras further reduces pancreatic FGF-21 increasing cancer propagation. High BMI, insulin resistance, and a high-fat diet contribute to increased insulin and visceral and intrapancreatic AT inflammation. AT-derived cytokine release and VAT stem cell translocation cause chronic pancreatic inflammation, including potentiation of Kras pathway. Changes in the gut microbiome cause pancreatic microbiome alterations, subsequently activating chronic inflammation via recruiting of M1 macrophages. Chronic fibroinflammatory changes lead to PanIN progression via NFkB pathway. Increased insulin and IGF-1 lead to stress granule formation that contributes to carcinogenesis via mTOR pathway independent of Kras pathway.

components leading to a systemic pro inflammatory state [77]. Certain lipopolysaccharides (LPS) producing bacteria alter the microbial profile in pancreas by reducing probiotics and butyrate-producing bacteria. LPS acts as a pro-inflammatory pro-tumor trigger by activating NFkB pathway which subsequently activates cytokines including IL-6, TNF, and IL-1. LPS excess could further lead to recruitment of proinflammatory M1-like macrophages, pancreatic fibrosis, chronic inflammation, and PanIN lesions [68, 74]. A positive feedback loop is initiated by amplification of Ras activity by NF-KB which triggers further inflammation and initiates a positive feedback loop found among oncogenic Ras activated mice [74].

2.6 Food carcinogens

Diet consisting of high grilled and fried meats, preservatives, some grains, and vegetables containing heterocyclic amines, aristolochic acids, polycyclic aromatic hydrocarbons, pyrrolizidine alkaloids, aflatoxins, acrylamide, N-nitroso compounds, and benzopyrenes have been positively associated with both obesity and PDAC in epidemiological studies [78–82]. An increased PC risk has been associated with higher exposure of these diets; however, evidence of temporal relationship and pathogenesis remains unclear. More recently, contradictory findings of deep-fried foods inversely related to risk of PDAC was found in prospective study (**Figure 1**) [83].

3. Implications in prevention

Epidemiology demonstrates obesity is one of the vital modifiable risk factors of PDAC [17–19]. Measures to combat obesity is therefore of utmost importance in prevention of this lethal cancer with delayed diagnosis, aggressive nature, and poor responses to current treatment options. At the national level, several strategies were implemented after the recognition of obesity as an epidemic. These include environmental changes, increase access to healthy foods, increasing fruit and vegetable intake, dietary approaches to stop hypertension (DASH) diet, encouraging breast-feeding, more physical activity for general health and cardiovascular disease prevention, and further focus on its role in PC prevention.

3.1 Calorie restriction

Animal models have shown calorie restriction slowed the PC growth and development. In a study using conditional KrasG12D mice, intermittent calorie restriction and chronic calorie restriction have shown a relatively lower percentage of PanIN3 lesions. Calorie restriction and diet modifications have been proven to reduce incidence of breast and endometrial cancers in observational studies. Efforts to combat obesity are increasingly identified. The biggest challenge is short-term weight loss occurs with calorie restriction and a vast majority of people cannot keep up and gain back the lost weight in the long term [55].

3.2 Bariatric surgery

A significant reduction in risk of PDAC and mortality was found in obese patients who underwent bariatric surgery consistently among several studies. Of note, 73% of patients in bariatric surgery arm were female and 79% were younger than 65 years of age. Relatively small sample size and short follow-up duration studies were unable to detect a significant difference in PC risk. Several mechanisms are proposed in its beneficial role in PDAC. A significant reduction of inflammatory markers (CRP, IL-6) activated T cells ratio and increased anti-inflammatory regulatory T cells in epididymal adipose tissues was noted as early as 3 weeks post-surgery [84]. Bariatric surgery significantly improved insulin resistance and improved intestinal microbiota profile with equal benefits with both Roux-en-Y gastric bypass and vertical banded gastroplasty [85]. Bariatric surgery provides a long term and durable weight loss than calorie restriction. At this time, overall survival rates in PDAC patients who underwent prior bariatric surgery are unclear.

3.3 Antidiabetic treatments

Metformin is implicated in reduction of PC risk by inhibition of cell growth, proliferation, migration, and cell invasion, however, is still not completely understood [39, 59–61, 86]. Inhibition of crosstalk of GPCR and insulin/IGFR pathway, activation of liver kinase B1 (LKB1), repurposing the adenosine monophosphate-activated protein kinase (AMPK) and ultimately the disruption of downstream mTOR pathway is a well-accepted mechanism [59, 87]. Metformin also downregulates the expression of YAP and TAZ in pancreas acinar cells in addition to reduction of insulin/IGF-1 levels [39, 61]. Mice studies have shown metformin in high-fat-fed mice normalized the obesity-induced gut dysbiosis and maintained higher levels of Akkermansia related to Clostridium sensu stricto microbiota which helps in maintaining a functioning gut barrier [75]. In an epidemiological meta-analysis, metformin reduced the risk to one-third compared to other diabetic treatments [88]. Metformin has shown significant survival benefits in patients among T2DM, early stage and resected PCs in contrast to metastatic stages where the benefits were unclear per a large meta-analysis [89, 90]. It is proposed that in the later stages, amount of metformin is relatively less in the tumor cells to show its fullest benefits owing from the observation that metformin showed increased survival rates among resected advanced-stage PDAC. Overall, current evidence has not proven metformin-associated survival benefits in PDAC. Given its well tolerability, a potential beneficial role in chemoprevention is favored rather than therapeutic setting. Metformin is not currently a part of guideline-based protocols. Randomized controlled trials are required to explore this further. Recent evidence has shown synergistic effects of aspirin and metformin in chemoprevention in PDAC by inhibition of COX and NFKB pathway in addition to mTOR pathway which might essentially benefit obese population [74, 91].

The idea of use of thiozolidiones and PPAR-gamma agonists navigated its way into experimental studies of PDAC prevention, as PPAR-gamma a vital regulator in cell differentiation and inflammation. In vitro studies demonstrated that PPAR-gamma agonists induce apoptosis, ductal differentiation, reduce cell motility, tissue invasion, and arrest in G0/G1 phase by PPAR-gamma dependent and independent mechanisms [92]. PPAR-gamma agonists also alter the total urokinase activity by reducing urokinase plasminogen activator, which is causally involved in PDAC pathogenesis, further studies are required for its use in therapeutic setting [30].

3.4 Anti-inflammatory agents

Mice studies demonstrated disruption of NFkB-mediated inflammatory pathway by decreasing the expression of NFkB kinase 2 or Cox-2. Interruption of the positive feedback loop by Cox-2 inhibitors is a potential preventive strategy among Ras-mediated cancers including pancreas, colon, and lung. This paved path for aspirin in PDAC and a synergistic effect with metformin, especially among obese patients [74]. However, an earlier prospective study of extended aspirin use showed statistically increased risk of PDAC among women [93]. Further studies are required for its validation.

3.5 Fibroblast growth factor-21 supplements

Normal pancreatic acinar cells express high levels of adipokine FGF-21 as described above. Among obese Kras mutated mice, FGF-21 levels were significantly low. In preclinical studies, FGF-21 injections have shown prevention of extensive inflammation, PanINs and PDAC among obese mice [48, 49]. FGF-21 might be used in chemoprevention and treatment of PDAC and requires further preclinical and clinical studies.

3.6 Beta-blockers and statins

Beta-blockers have come into focus in PDAC chemoprevention by its effects on downregulation of cAMP-dependent endothelin growth factor (EGF) and vaso endothelin (VEGF) production. Statins are being evaluated in PDAC prevention by its effects of inhibition of 3 hydroxy3 methylglutaryl coenzyme A (HMGcoA) reductase effects on degradation of TP53 and reduced Ras activity. However, these agents have not been studied in relation to obesity-associated PDAC [86].

3.7 Screening

Currently, no screening guidelines exist for PDAC in high-risk obesity. Computed tomography (CT) screening was evaluated in T2DM at the time of diagnosis, however, has not reached evidence of significance. A predefined elevated IGF-1/IGFBP-3 ratio could be used as a screening tool to identify high-risk obesity patients. It is possible to identify prediction models based on epigenomic, transcriptomic, and proteomic approaches for obesity-driven carcinogenesis using appropriate in vitro and in vivo models that may be used for early detection of PDAC in obese high-risk individuals [29].

4. Implications in treatment

Surgery remains the mainstay for curative intent. However, at presentation, only 15–20% of PDAC are resectable. For locally advanced unresectable and metastatic PDACs, palliative systemic therapy including combinational chemotherapy has shown improvement in disease-related symptoms and prolonged survival. Genetic testing is recommended in all newly diagnosed PDAC patients and molecular testing for mutations in metastatic setting. Currently, we have limited treatment options beyond first line therapies. Treatment choices must be weighed against best supportive care.

4.1 Targeted agents

At this time, there are limited targeted therapy options in PDAC outside of clinical trials. Currently, targeted options are approved for BReast CAncer gene (BRCA) 1/2 mutations (olaparib), Microsatellite Instability (MSI) high (pembrolizumab),

Neurotrophic tyrosine receptor kinase (NTRK) mutations (entrectinib, Larotrectinib), and B-Rapidly Accelerated Fibrosarcoma (BRAF) V600E mutations (Dabrafenib+ Trametinib) [94–98]. Although Kras mutations are major drivers of PDAC, several decades of research has not been able to find a targeted therapy against Kras due to its high affinity for GTP activity and absence of an amenable surface topologic target [33]. As a result, past efforts have mainly focused on indirect strategies to target the downstream signals. Recent success in identifying small molecules that directly bind to RAS, has fueled hope that RAS may be druggable after all. Sotorasib, a KrasG12C inhibitor traps Kras in the inactive GDP-bound conformational state by fitting tightly into a unique phosphate binding pocket and is recently FDA approved. A phase 1/2 trial, CodeBreak100 (NCT03600883), demonstrated that 8/38 (21%) patients had confirmed partial responses and 32/38 (84%) patients had disease control in a median follow-up of 16.8 months. Only 1–2% of PDAC patients have KrasG12C mutations and its inhibitor is clinically meaningful in these cases [99, 100]. Currently, there are ongoing trials for KrasG12D siRNA-targeted therapies (NCT03608631). Understanding pathogenesis of obesity-driven PDAC could potentially recognize further therapeutic targets. Several studies in preclinical settings are ongoing for targeting various steps in the pathogenesis of PDAC. One such example is blocking the downstream step of SG formation. Hyperactivation of IGF-1/PI3K/mTOR/S6K1 pathway leads to SRPK2-mediated SG formation, a vital step in obesity-associated PDAC. S6K1 inhibition selectively attenuates IGF-1-driven SGs formation and can potentially be a treatment target [58].

4.2 Future perspectives for adjunctive therapies

Strategies for microbiome modification or other options could potentially control metabolic endotoxemia as an adjunctive treatment of PDAC remains unknown [70].

4.3 Exercise interventions

Individualized exercise interventions are increasingly identified as effective therapy as an adjunct in PDAC management, improving quality and quantity of life, reducing treatment side effects, enhancing fitness preoperatively, combating cancer-related fatigue, and overall psychological health benefits [101–103]. Aerobic and resistance exercise reduced symptoms of depression and anxiety in all PDAC stages and settings, in line with other common cancers such as breast cancer [103, 104]. Exercise regimens tailored to improve skeletal muscle health preoperatively and in neoadjuvant settings has shown to improve clinical and quality of life outcomes [101, 105]. The feasibility of multimodal cachexia intervention with resistance training, nutritional supplements, and anti-inflammatory agents such as celecoxib was tested in PDAC-related cachexia. These modalities have cleared the safety threshold and compliance goals. Currently, phase II studies are underway to test the efficacy [106, 107]. A systematic review that looked at overall exercise effects did not show any adverse effects related to exercise in PDAC patients. However, limitation includes a smaller sample size and finite data from case reports/studies. Overall results supported safety and feasibility of exercise training in PDAC patients [103]. The underlying mechanism of this benefit remains unclear. Due to the high burden of disease and treatment-related adverse effects, exercise compliance also is a major challenge for PDAC patients. Individualized regular exercise regimens and shorter assessment intervals are required to evaluate the short-term benefits of exercise in a disease which has shorter life expectancy.

5. Conclusion

Obesity is a major independent and modifiable risk factor of PDAC. The biological link between obesity and PDAC is complex and convoluted. The interplay is driven by genetic, hormonal factors, insulin resistance, adipokines, circulating lipids, and gut microbiome dysbiosis. These findings indicate that there is unlikely to be a single mechanism to explain obesity-associated PDAC. Awareness and deeper knowledge could help implement potential preventive measures (diet modifications, exercise, and bariatric surgeries) and treatment modalities. Prospective trials to evaluate metformin in chemoprevention, screening in high-risk obese populations, risk predictive models, KrasG12D directed therapies, adjunct use of gut microbiota transplantation, and personalized therapies are some future perspectives.

Conflict of interest

The authors declare no conflict of interest.

List of abbreviations

PDAC	pancreatic ductal adenocarcinoma
Kras	Kirsten Rat Sarcoma viral oncogene
US	United States
PC	pancreatic cancer
IRR	incidence risk ratio
BMI	body mass index
WC	waist circumference
WHR	waist-hip ratio
CDC	Centers for Disease Control
COVID19	Coronavirus Disease 2019
RR	relative risk
CI	confidence interval
MCN	mucinous cystic neoplasms
IPMN	intraductal papillary mucinous neoplasms
PanIN	pancreatic intraepithelial neoplasms
IGF1	insulin-like growth factor 1
MEK	mitogen-activated protein kinase
ERK	extracellular signal-regulated kinase
AT	adipose tissue
LCN-2	lipocalin-2
FGF-21	fibroblast growth factor
Wnt5a	wingless-type mouse mammary tumor virus integration site family member 5A
Sfrp-5	secreted frizzled-related protein
VAT	visceral adipose tissue
YAP	yes-associated protein
IL	interleukin
TNF	tumor necrosis factor
T2DM	type 2 diabetes mellitus

IGFBP	insulin growth factor binding proteins
GPCR	G protein coupled receptors
TAZ	PDZ binding motif
SG	stress granules
S6K	S6 kinase
SRPK	serine/arginine protein kinase
Th	T helper
NK	natural killer
MHC	major histocompatibility complex
IFN	interferon
NFkB	nuclear factor kappa B
PPAR-gamma	peroxisome proliferator-activated receptor-gamma
LPS	liposaccharides
DASH	dietary approaches to stop hypertension
LKB1	liver kinase B1
AMPK	adenosine monophosphate-activated protein kinase
EGF	endothelin growth factor
VEGF	vaso endothelin growth factor
HMGcoA	3 hydroxy 3 methylglutaryl coenzyme A
CT	computed tomography
BRCA	BReast CAncer gene
MSI	microsatellite instability
NTRK	neurotrophic tyrosine receptor kinase
BRAF	B rapidly accelerated fibrosarcoma

Appendices and nomenclature

None.

Author details

Nikitha Vobugari and Kai Sun*
Department of Hematology/Oncology, Houston Methodist Hospital, Houston, TX, USA

*Address all correspondence to: ksun2@houstonmethodist.org

References

[1] Ali H, Pamarthy R, Vallabhaneni M, Sarfraz S, Ali H, Rafique H. Pancreatic cancer incidence trends in the United States from 2000-2017: Analysis of Surveillance, Epidemiology and End Results (SEER) database [version 1; peer review: 2 approved]. F1000Research. 2021;**10**:529. DOI: 10.12688/f1000research.54390.1

[2] Moshayedi N, Escobedo AL, Thomassian S, Osipov A, Hendifar AE. Race, sex, age, and geographic disparities in pancreatic cancer incidence. Journal of Clinical Oncology. 2022;**40**(4_suppl):520

[3] McWilliams RR, Maisonneuve P, Bamlet WR, Petersen GM, Li D, Risch HA, et al. Risk factors for early-onset and very-early-onset pancreatic adenocarcinoma: A Pancreatic Cancer Case-Control Consortium (PanC4) Analysis. Pancreas. 2016;**45**(2):311-316

[4] Wu W, He X, Yang L, Wang Q, Bian X, Ye J, et al. Rising trends in pancreatic cancer incidence and mortality in 2000-2014. Clinical Epidemiology. 2018;**10**:789-797

[5] Sung H, Ferlay J, Siegel RL, Laversanne M, Soerjomataram I, Jemal A, et al. Global cancer statistics 2020: GLOBOCAN estimates of incidence and mortality worldwide for 36 cancers in 185 countries. CA: a Cancer Journal for Clinicians. 2021;**71**(3):209-249

[6] Jemal A, Siegel R, Xu J, Ward E. Cancer statistics, 2010. CA: a Cancer Journal for Clinicians. 2010;**60**(5):277-300

[7] American Cancer Society. Cancer facts & figures. Atlanta American Cancer Society. 2022;**2022**:1-80

[8] Hu JX, Lin YY, Zhao CF, Chen WB, Liu QC, Li QW, et al. Pancreatic cancer: A review of epidemiology, trend, and risk factors. World Journal of Gastroenterology. 2021;**27**(27):4298-4321

[9] Flegal KM, Carroll MD, Ogden CL, Johnson CL. Prevalence and trends in obesity among US adults, 1999-2000. Journal of the American Medical Association. 2002;**288**(14):1723-1727

[10] Physical status: The use and interpretation of anthropometry. World Health Organization Technical Report Series. 1995;**854**:1-452. PMID: 8594834

[11] Garrow JS, Webster J. Quetelet's index (W/H2) as a measure of fatness. International Journal of Obesity. 1985;**9**(2):147-153

[12] Stierman B, Afful J, Carroll MD, Chen TC, Davy O, Fink S, et al. National health and nutrition examination survey 2017–March 2020 prepandemic data files-development of files and prevalence estimates for selected health outcomes. National Health Statistics Reports. 2021;**2021**(158). DOI: 10.15620/cdc:106273

[13] Dietz WH. The response of the US Centers for Disease Control and Prevention to the obesity epidemic. Annual Review of Public Health. 2015;**36**:575-596

[14] Restrepo BJ. Obesity prevalence among U.S. adults during the COVID-19 pandemic. American Journal of Preventive Medicine. 2022;**63**(1):102-106

[15] U.S. Cancer Statistics Working Group. U.S. Cancer Statistics Data Visualizations Tool, Based on 2021 Submission Data (1999-2019). U.S.

Department of Health and Human Services, Centers for Disease Control and Prevention and National Cancer Institute; 2022 Available from: https://gis.cdc.gov/Cancer/USCS/#/RiskFactors/

[16] Davoodi SH, Malek-Shahabi T, Malekshahi-Moghadam A, Shahbazi R, Esmaeili S. Obesity as an important risk factor for certain types of cancer. Iranian Journal of Cancer Prevention. 2013;**6**(4):186-194

[17] Arslan AA, Helzlsouer KJ, Kooperberg C, Shu XO, Steplowski E, Bueno-De-Mesquita HB, et al. Anthropometric measures, body mass index, and pancreatic cancer: A pooled analysis from the pancreatic cancer cohort consortium (PanScan). Archives of Internal Medicine. 2010;**170**(9):791-802

[18] Jiao L, Berrington De Gonzalez A, Hartge P, Pfeiffer RM, Park Y, Freedman DM, et al. Body mass index, effect modifiers, and risk of pancreatic cancer: A pooled study of seven prospective cohorts. Cancer Causes & Control. 2010;**21**(8):1305-1314

[19] Renehan AG, Tyson M, Egger M, Heller RF, Zwahlen M. Body-mass index and incidence of cancer: A systematic review and meta-analysis of prospective observational studies. Lancet. 2008;**371**(9612):569-578

[20] Aune D, Greenwood DC, Chan DSM, Vieira R, Vieira AR, Navarro Rosenblatt DA, et al. Body mass index, abdominal fatness and pancreatic cancer risk: A systematic review and non-linear dose-response meta-analysis of prospective studies. Annals of Oncology. 2012;**23**(4):843-852

[21] Kasenda B, Bass A, Koeberle D, Pestalozzi B, Borner M, Herrmann R, et al. Survival in overweight patients with advanced pancreatic carcinoma: A multicentre cohort study. BMC Cancer. 29 Sep 2014;**14**(1):728. DOI: 10.1186/1471-2407-14-728. PMID: 25266049; PMCID: PMC4242603

[22] Li D, Morris JS, Liu J, Hassan MM, Day RS, Bondy ML, et al. Body mass index and risk, age of onset, and survival in patients with pancreatic cancer. JAMA. 2009;**301**(24):2553-2562

[23] Johansen D, Stocks T, Jonsson H, Lindkvist B, Björge T, Concin H, et al. Metabolic factors and the risk of pancreatic cancer: A prospective analysis of almost 580,000 men and women in the metabolic syndrome and cancer project. Cancer Epidemiology, Biomarkers & Prevention. 2010;**19**(9):2307-2317

[24] Genkinger JM, Spiegelman D, Anderson KE, Bernstein L, Van Den Brandt PA, Calle EE, et al. A pooled analysis of 14 cohort studies of anthropometric factors and pancreatic cancer risk. International Journal of Cancer. 2011;**129**(7):1708-1717

[25] Zohar L, Rottenberg Y, Twig G, Katz L, Leiba A, Derazne E, et al. Adolescent overweight and obesity and the risk for pancreatic cancer among men and women: A nationwide study of 1.79 million Israeli adolescents. Cancer. 2019;**125**(1):118-126

[26] Silverman DT, Swanson CA, Gridley G, Wacholder S, Greenberg RS, Brown LM, et al. Dietary and nutritional factors and pancreatic cancer: A case-control study based on direct interviews. Journal of the National Cancer Institute. 1998;**90**(22):1710-1719

[27] Genkinger JM, Kitahara CM, Bernstein L, Berrington de Gonzalez A, Brotzman M, Elena JW, et al. Central adiposity, obesity during early adulthood, and pancreatic cancer

mortality in a pooled analysis of cohort studies. Annals of Oncology. 2015;**26**(11):2257-2266

[28] Calle EE, Rodriguez C, Walker-Thurmond K, Thun MJ. Overweight, obesity, and mortality from cancer in a prospectively studied cohort of U.S. Adults. The New England Journal of Medicine. 2003;**348**(17):1625-1638

[29] Kfoury S, Michl P, Roth L. Modeling obesity-driven pancreatic carcinogenesis—A review of current in vivo and in vitro models of obesity and pancreatic carcinogenesis. Cell. 10 Oct 2022;**11**(19):3170. DOI: 10.3390/cells11193170. PMID: 36231132; PMCID: PMC9563584

[30] Polvani S, Tarocchi M, Tempesti S, Bencini L, Galli A. Peroxisome proliferator activated receptors at the crossroad of obesity, diabetes, and pancreatic cancer. World Journal of Gastroenterology. 2016;**22**(8):2441-2459

[31] Pisani P. Hyper-insulinaemia and cancer, meta-analyses of epidemiological studies. Archives of Physiology and Biochemistry. 2008;**114**(1):63-70

[32] Eibl G, Rozengurt E. Obesity and pancreatic cancer: Insight into mechanisms. Cancers (Basel). 10 Oct 2021;**13**(20):5067. DOI: 10.3390/cancers13205067. PMID: 34680216; PMCID: PMC8534007

[33] Waters AM, Der CJ. KRAS: The critical driver and therapeutic target for pancreatic cancer. Cold Spring Harbor Perspectives in Medicine. 4 Sep 2018;**8**(9):a031435. DOI: 10.1101/cshperspect.a031435. PMID: 29229669; PMCID: PMC5995645

[34] Hingorani SR, Petricoin EF, Maitra A, Rajapakse V, King C, Jacobetz MA, et al. Preinvasive and invasive ductal pancreatic cancer and its early detection in the mouse. Cancer Cell. 2003;**4**(6):437-450

[35] Notta F, Hahn SA, Real FX. A genetic roadmap of pancreatic cancer: Still evolving. Gut. 2017;**66**(12):2170-2178

[36] Iacobuzio-Donahue CA. Genetic evolution of pancreatic cancer: Lessons learnt from the pancreatic cancer genome sequencing project. Gut. 2012;**61**(7):1085-1094

[37] Dawson DW, Hertzer K, Moro A, Donald G, Chang HH, Go VL, et al. High-fat, high-calorie diet promotes early pancreatic neoplasia in the conditional KrasG12D mouse model. Cancer Prevention Research. 2013;**6**(10):1064-1073

[38] Eibl G, Rozengurt E. KRAS, YAP, and obesity in pancreatic cancer: A signaling network with multiple loops. Seminars in Cancer Biology. 2019;**54**:50-62

[39] Chang HH, Moro A, Chou CEN, Dawson DW, French S, Schmidt AI, et al. Metformin decreases the incidence of pancreatic ductal adenocarcinoma promoted by diet-induced obesity in the conditional KrasG12D Mouse Model. Scientific Reports. 12 Apr 2018;**8**(1):5899. DOI: 10.1038/s41598-018-24337-8. PMID: 29651002; PMCID: PMC5897574

[40] Bracci PM. Obesity and pancreatic cancer: Overview of epidemiologic evidence and biologic mechanisms. Molecular Carcinogenesis. 2012;**51**(1):53-63

[41] Izquierdo AG, Crujeiras AB, Casanueva FF, Carreira MC. Leptin, obesity, and leptin resistance: Where are we 25 years later? Nutrients. 8 Nov 2019;**11**(11):2704. DOI: 10.3390/nu11112704. PMID: 31717265; PMCID: PMC6893721

[42] Friedman J. The long road to leptin. The Journal of Clinical Investigation. 2016;**126**(12):4727-4734

[43] Bao Y, Giovannucci EL, Kraft P, Stampfer MJ, Ogino S, Ma J, et al. A prospective study of plasma adiponectin and pancreatic cancer risk in five US cohorts. Journal of the National Cancer Institute. 2013;**105**(2):95-103

[44] Dranka-Bojarowska D, Lekstan A, Olakowski M, Jablonska B, Lewinski A, Musialski P, et al. The assessment of serum concentration of adiponectin, leptin and serum carbohydrate antigen-19.9 in patients with pancreatic cancer and chronic pancreatitis. Journal of Physiology and Pharmacology. 2015;**66**(5):653-663

[45] Moniaux N, Chakraborty S, Yalniz M, Gonzalez J, Shostrom VK, Standop J, et al. Early diagnosis of pancreatic cancer: Neutrophil gelatinase-associated lipocalin as a marker of pancreatic intraepithelial neoplasia. British Journal of Cancer. 2008;**98**(9):1540-1547

[46] Xu B, Jin DY, Lou WH, Wang DS. Lipocalin-2 is associated with a good prognosis and reversing epithelial-to-mesenchymal transition in pancreatic cancer. World Journal of Surgery. 2013;**37**(8):1892-1900

[47] Tong Z, Kunnumakkara AB, Wang H, Matsuo Y, Diagaradjane P, Harikumar KB, et al. Neutrophil gelatinase-associated lipocalin: A novel suppressor of invasion and angiogenesis in pancreatic cancer. Cancer Research. 2008;**68**(15):6100-6108

[48] Lu W, Li X, Luo Y. FGF21 in obesity and cancer: New insights. Cancer Letters. 2021;**499**:5-13

[49] Luo Y, Yang Y, Liu M, Wang D, Wang F, Bi Y, et al. Oncogenic KRAS reduces expression of FGF21 in acinar cells to promote pancreatic tumorigenesis in mice on a high-fat diet. Gastroenterology. 2019;**157**(5): 1413-1428.e11

[50] Tu B, Yao J, Ferri-Borgogno S, Zhao J, Chen S, Wang Q, et al. YAP1 oncogene is a context-specific driver for pancreatic ductal adenocarcinoma. JCI. Insight. 2019;**4**(21)

[51] Ouchi N, Parker JL, Lugus JJ, Walsh K. Adipokines in inflammation and metabolic disease. Nature Reviews. Immunology. Feb 2011;**11**(2):85-97. DOI: 10.1038/nri2921. Epub 2011 Jan 21. PMID: 21252989; PMCID: PMC3518031

[52] Crewe C, Funcke JB, Li S, Joffin N, Gliniak CM, Ghaben AL, et al. Extracellular vesicle-based interorgan transport of mitochondria from energetically stressed adipocytes. Cell Metabolism. 2021;**33**(9):1853-1868.e11

[53] Rebours V, Gaujoux S, D' Assignies G, Sauvanet A, Ruszniewski P, Lévy P, et al. Obesity and fatty pancreatic infiltration are risk factors for pancreatic precancerous lesions (PanIN). Clinical Cancer Research. 2015;**21**(15):3522-3528

[54] Hertzer KM, Xu M, Moro A, Dawson DW, Du L, Li G, et al. Robust early inflammation of the peripancreatic visceral adipose tissue during diet-induced obesity in the KRASG12D model of pancreatic cancer. Pancreas. 2016;**45**(3):458-465

[55] Xu M, Jung X, Hines OJ, Eibl G, Chen Y. Obesity and pancreatic cancer: Overview of epidemiology and potential prevention by weight loss. Pancreas. 2018;**47**(2):158-162

[56] Sreedhar UL, DeSouza SV, Park B, Petrov MS. A systematic review of intra-pancreatic fat deposition and pancreatic carcinogenesis.

Journal of Gastrointestinal Surgery. 2020;**24**(11):2560-2569

[57] Abbruzzese JL, Andersen DK, Borrebaeck CAK, Chari ST, Costello E, Cruz-Monserrate Z, et al. The interface of pancreatic cancer with diabetes, obesity, and inflammation: Research gaps and opportunities: Summary of a national Institute of Diabetes and digestive and kidney diseases workshop. Pancreas. 2018;**47**(5):516-525

[58] Fonteneau G, Redding A, Hoag-Lee H, Sim ES, Heinrich S, Gaida MM, et al. Stress granules determine the development of obesity-associated pancreatic cancer. Cancer Discovery. 2022;**12**(8):1984-2005

[59] Kisfalvi K, Eibl G, Sinnett-Smith J, Rozengurt E. Metformin disrupts crosstalk between G protein-coupled receptor and insulin receptor signaling systems and inhibits pancreatic cancer growth. Cancer Research. 2009;**69**(16):6539-6545

[60] Rozengurt E, Sinnett-Smith J, Kisfalvi K. Crosstalk between insulin/insulin-like growth factor-1 receptors and G protein-coupled receptor signaling systems: A novel target for the antidiabetic drug metformin in pancreatic cancer. Clinical Cancer Research. 2010;**16**(9):2505-2511

[61] Rozengurt E, Eibl G. Central role of Yes-associated protein and WW-domain-containing transcriptional co-activator with PDZ-binding motif in pancreatic cancer development. World Journal of Gastroenterology. 2019;**25**(15):1797-1816

[62] Douglas JB, Silverman DT, Pollak MN, Tao Y, Soliman AS, Stolzenberg-Solomon RZ. Serum IGF-I, IGF-II, IGFBP-3, and IGF-I/IGFBP-3 molar ratio and risk of pancreatic cancer in the prostate, lung, colorectal, and ovarian cancer screening trial. Cancer Epidemiology, Biomarkers & Prevention. 2010;**19**(9):2298-2306

[63] Garay-Sevilla ME, Gomez-Ojeda A, González I, Luévano-Contreras C, Rojas A. Contribution of RAGE axis activation to the association between metabolic syndrome and cancer. Molecular and Cellular Biochemistry. 2021;**476**(3):1555-1573

[64] Polvani S, Tarocchi M, Tempesti S, Galli A. Nuclear receptors and pathogenesis of pancreatic cancer. World Journal of Gastroenterology. 2014;**20**(34):12062-12081

[65] Chan KS, Ho BCS, Shelat VG. A pilot study of estrogen receptor (ER) expression in pancreatic ductal adenocarcinoma (PDAC). Translational Gastroenterology and Hepatology. 5 Jan 2021;**6**:9. DOI: 10.21037/tgh.2020.02.16. PMID: 33409403; PMCID: PMC7724184

[66] Seeliger H, Pozios I, Assmann G, Zhao Y, Müller MH, Knösel T, et al. Expression of estrogen receptor beta correlates with adverse prognosis in resected pancreatic adenocarcinoma. BMC Cancer. 29 Oct 2018;**18**(1):1049. DOI: 10.1186/s12885-018-4973-6. PMID: 30373552; PMCID: PMC6206939

[67] Martinez-Santibañez G, Cho KW, Lumeng CN. Imaging white adipose tissue with confocal microscopy. Methods in Enzymology. 2014;**537**:17-30

[68] Teper Y, Eibl G. Pancreatic macrophages: Critical players in obesity-promoted pancreatic cancer. Cancers (Basel). 2020;**12**(7):1-16

[69] Deng T, Lyon CJ, Bergin S, Caligiuri MA, Hsueh WA. Obesity, inflammation, and cancer. Annual Review of Pathology: Mechanisms of Disease. 2016;**11**:421-449

[70] Cani PD, Bibiloni R, Knauf C, Waget A, Neyrinck AM, Delzenne NM,

et al. Changes in gut microbiota control metabolic endotoxemia-induced inflammation in high-fat diet-induced obesity and diabetes in mice. Diabetes. 2008;**57**(6):1470-1481

[71] Chen J, Pitmon E, Wang K. Microbiome, inflammation and colorectal cancer. Seminars in Immunology. 2017;**32**:43-53

[72] Yoshimoto S, Loo TM, Atarashi K, Kanda H, Sato S, Oyadomari S, et al. Obesity-induced gut microbial metabolite promotes liver cancer through senescence secretome. Nature. 2013;**499**(7456):97-101

[73] Thomas RM, Gharaibeh RZ, Gauthier J, Beveridge M, Pope JL, Guijarro MV, et al. Intestinal microbiota enhances pancreatic carcinogenesis in preclinical models. Carcinogenesis. 2018;**39**(8):1068-1078

[74] Daniluk J, Liu Y, Deng D, Chu J, Huang H, Gaiser S, et al. An NF-κB pathway-mediated positive feedback loop amplifies Ras activity to pathological levels in mice. The Journal of Clinical Investigation. 2012;**122**(4):1519-1528

[75] Dong TS, Chang HH, Hauer M, Lagishetty V, Katzka W, Rozengurt E, et al. Metformin alters the duodenal microbiome and decreases the incidence of pancreatic ductal adenocarcinoma promoted by diet-induced obesity. American Journal of Physiology. Gastrointestinal and Liver Physiology. 2019;**317**(6):G763-G772

[76] Dao MC, Everard A, Aron-Wisnewsky J, Sokolovska N, Prifti E, Verger EO, et al. Akkermansia muciniphila and improved metabolic health during a dietary intervention in obesity: Relationship with gut microbiome richness and ecology. Gut. 2016;**65**(3):426-436

[77] Boutagy NE, McMillan RP, Frisard MI, Hulver MW. Metabolic endotoxemia with obesity: Is it real and is it relevant? Biochimie. 2016;**124**:11-20

[78] Anderson KE, Kadlubar FF, Kulldorff M, Harnack L, Gross M, Lang NP, et al. Dietary intake of heterocyclic amines and benzo(a)pyrene: Associations with pancreatic cancer. Cancer Epidemiology, Biomarkers & Prevention. 2005;**14**(9):2261-2265

[79] Li D, Day RS, Bondy ML, Sinha R, Nguyen NT, Evans DB, et al. Dietary mutagen exposure and risk of pancreatic cancer. Cancer Epidemiology, Biomarkers & Prevention. 2007;**16**(4):655-661

[80] Anderson KE, Sinha R, Kulldorff M, Gross M, Lang NP, Barber C, et al. Meat intake and cooking techniques: Associations with pancreatic cancer. Mutation Research, Fundamental and Molecular Mechanisms of Mutagenesis. 2002;**506-507**:225-231

[81] Stolzenberg-Solomon RZ, Cross AJ, Silverman DT, Schairer C, Thompson FE, Kipnis V, et al. Meat and meat-mutagen intake and pancreatic cancer risk in the NIH-AARP cohort. Cancer Epidemiology, Biomarkers & Prevention. 2007;**16**(12):2664-2675

[82] Kobets T, Smith BPC, Williams GM. Food-borne chemical carcinogens and the evidence for human cancer risk. Food. 2022;**11**(18):88-100

[83] Zhong GC, Zhu Q, Gong JP, Cai D, Hu JJ, Dai X, et al. Fried food consumption and the risk of pancreatic cancer: A large prospective multicenter study. Frontiers in Nutrition. 22 Jul 2022;**9**:889303. DOI: 10.3389/fnut.2022.889303. PMID: 35958255; PMCID: PMC9362838

[84] Schneck AS, Iannelli A, Patouraux S, Rousseau D, Bonnafous S,

Bailly-Maitre B, et al. Effects of sleeve gastrectomy in high fat diet-induced obese mice: Respective role of reduced caloric intake, whiteadipose tissue inflammation and changes in adipose tissue and ectopic fat depots. Surgical Endoscopy. 2014;**28**(2):592-602

[85] Tremaroli V, Karlsson F, Werling M, Ståhlman M, Kovatcheva-Datchary P, Olbers T, et al. Roux-en-Y gastric bypass and vertical banded gastroplasty induce long-term changes on the human gut microbiome contributing to fat mass regulation. Cell Metabolism. 2015;**22**(2):228-238

[86] Miyaki C, Lynch LM. An update on common pharmaceuticals in the prevention of pancreatic cancer. Cureus. 30 May 2022;**14**(5):e25496. DOI: 10.7759/cureus.25496. PMID: 35800820; PMCID: PMC9246430

[87] Sinnett-Smith J, Kisfalvi K, Kui R, Rozengurt E. Metformin inhibition of mTORC1 activation, DNA synthesis and proliferation in pancreatic cancer cells: Dependence on glucose concentration and role of AMPK. Biochemical and Biophysical Research Communications. 2013;**430**(1):352-357

[88] Wang Z, Lai S t, Xie L, Dong ZJ, Yi MN, Zhu J, et al. Metformin is associated with reduced risk of pancreatic cancer in patients with type 2 diabetes mellitus: A systematic review and meta-analysis. Diabetes Research and Clinical Practice. 2014;**106**(1):19-26

[89] Li X, Li T, Liu Z, Gou S, Wang C. The effect of metformin on survival of patients with pancreatic cancer: A meta-analysis. Scientific Reports. 19 Jul 2017;**7**(1):5825. DOI: 10.1038/s41598-017-06207-x. PMID: 28724893; PMCID: PMC5517652

[90] Zhou PT, Li B, Liu FR, Zhang MC, Wang Q, Li YY, et al. Metformin is associated with survival benefit in pancreatic cancer patients with diabetes: A systematic review and metaanalysis. Oncotarget. 2017;**8**(15):25242-25250

[91] Yue W, Yang CS, DiPaola RS, Tan XL. Repurposing of metformin and aspirin by targeting AMPK-mTOR and inflammation for pancreatic cancer prevention and treatment. Cancer Prevention Research. 2014;**7**(4):388-397

[92] Hong J, Samudio I, Liu S, Abdelrahim M, Safe S. Peroxisome proliferator-activated receptor γ-dependent activation of p21 in Panc-28 pancreatic cancer cells involves Sp1 and Sp4 proteins. Endocrinology. 2004;**145**(12):5774-5785

[93] Schernhammer ES, Kang JH, Chan AT, Michaud DS, Skinner HG, Giovannucci E, et al. A prospective study of aspirin use and the risk of pancreatic cancer in women. Journal of the National Cancer Institute. 2004;**96**(1):22-28

[94] Salama AKS, Li S, Macrae ER, Park JI, Mitchell EP, Zwiebel JA, et al. Dabrafenib and trametinib in patients with tumors with BRAFV600E mutations: Results of the NCI-MATCH trial subprotocol H. Journal of Clinical Oncology. 2020;**38**(33):3895-3904

[95] Marabelle A, Le DT, Ascierto PA, Di Giacomo AM, de Jesus-Acosta A, Delord JP, et al. Efficacy of pembrolizumab in patients with noncolorectal high microsatellite instability/ mismatch repair–deficient cancer: Results from the phase II KEYNOTE-158 study. Journal of Clinical Oncology. 2020;**38**(1):1-10

[96] Hammel P, Vitellius C, Boisteau É, Wisniewski M, Colle E, Hilmi M, et al. Maintenance therapies in metastatic pancreatic cancer: Present and future with a focus

on PARP inhibitors. Therapeutic Advances in Medical Oncology. 9 Jul 2020;**12**:1758835920937949. DOI: 10.1177/1758835920937949. PMID: 32695234; PMCID: PMC7350045

[97] Wang S, Zheng Y, Yang F, Zhu L, Zhu XQ, Wang ZF, et al. The molecular biology of pancreatic adenocarcinoma: Translational challenges and clinical perspectives. Signal Transduction and Targeted Therapy. 5 Jul 2021;**6**(1):249. DOI: 10.1038/s41392-021-00659-4. PMID: 34219130; PMCID: PMC8255319

[98] Sohal DPS, Kennedy EB, Cinar P, Conroy T, Copur MS, Crane CH, et al. Metastatic pancreatic cancer: ASCO guideline update. Journal of Clinical Oncology. 2020;**38**(27):3217-3230

[99] Hong DS, Fakih MG, Strickler JH, Desai J, Durm GA, Shapiro GI, et al. KRAS G12C inhibition with sotorasib in advanced solid tumors. The New England Journal of Medicine. 2020;**383**(13):1207-1217

[100] Strickler JH, Satake H, Hollebecque A, Sunakawa Y, Tomasini P, Bajor DL, et al. First data for sotorasib in patients with pancreatic cancer with KRAS p.G12C mutation: A phase I/II study evaluating efficacy and safety. Journal of Clinical Oncology. 2022;**40**(36_suppl):360490

[101] Singh F, Newton RU, Galvão DA, Spry N, Baker MK. A systematic review of pre-surgical exercise intervention studies with cancer patients. Surgical Oncology. 2013;**22**(2):92-104

[102] Speck RM, Courneya KS, Mâsse LC, Duval S, Schmitz KH. An update of controlled physical activity trials in cancer survivors: A systematic review and meta-analysis. Journal of Cancer Survivorship. 2010;**4**(2):87-100

[103] Luo H, Galvão DA, Newton RU, Lopez P, Tang C, Fairman CM, et al. Exercise medicine in the management of pancreatic cancer: A systematic review. Pancreas. 2021;**50**(3):280-292

[104] Cormie P, Spry N, Jasas K, Johansson M, Yusoff IF, Newton RU, et al. Exercise as medicine in the management of pancreatic cancer: A case study. Medicine and Science in Sports and Exercise. 2014;**46**(4):664-670

[105] Parker NH, Gorzelitz J, Ngo-Huang A, Caan BJ, Prakash L, Garg N, et al. The role of home-based exercise in maintaining skeletal muscle during preoperative pancreatic cancer treatment. Integrative Cancer Therapies. Jan-Dec 2021;**20**:1534735420986615. DOI: 10.1177/1534735420986615. PMID: 33870744; PMCID: PMC8056559

[106] Solheim TS, Laird BJA, Balstad TR, Stene GB, Bye A, Johns N, et al. A randomized phase II feasibility trial of a multimodal intervention for the management of cachexia in lung and pancreatic cancer. Journal of Cachexia, Sarcopenia and Muscle. 2017;**8**(5):778-788

[107] Naito T, Mitsunaga S, Miura S, Tatematsu N, Inano T, Mouri T, et al. Feasibility of early multimodal interventions for elderly patients with advanced pancreatic and non-small-cell lung cancer. Journal of Cachexia, Sarcopenia and Muscle. 2019;**10**(1):73-83

Chapter 3

Epidemiology and Risk Factors of Pancreatic Cancer

Michele Molinari, Hao Liu and Christof Kaltenmeier

Abstract

Pancreatic cancer (PC) is among the most common tumors of the gastrointestinal system in the world. In the United States and in other industrialized countries, it represents the fourth leading cause of cancer-related mortality. The incidence of PC increases with age and most patients are diagnosed after the age of 50. The overall prognosis of PC is poor. Most tumors are silent and they often present when metastatic. Only less than 15% of patients can undergo surgery, which represents the only potential cure for PC, and less than 10% of patients are alive after 5 years. In this chapter, we present the epidemiology of PC and its most common risk factors.

Keywords: pancreatic cancer, risk factors, epidemiology, screening for pancreatic cancer, nutritional status and pancreatic cancer

1. Introduction

Worldrwide, pancreatic cancer (PC) is the 12th most common cancer [1] and the fourth leading cause of cancer-related mortality in the United States with estimated 42,500 new cases and 35,000 deaths each year [2] (**Figure 1**). The age-standardized incidence of PC is 4.9 per 100,000 individuals [1] (**Figure 2**). There are significant variations in the incidence of PC among different geographical areas (**Figure 3**). In high-income countries, the incidence of PC is much higher than in low-income countries (11 vs. 3 per 100,000 individuals). PC ranks fifth after colorectal cancer, gastric cancer, hepatic cancer, and esophageal cancer among all gastrointestinal malignancies [3] (**Table 1**). Over time, the mortality rate for males has decreased by 0.4% while the mortality rate for females has increased by 4.4% [2]. More than 80% of PCs are diagnosed in patients older than 60 and almost 50% have distant metastases at the time of their clinical presentation [3–5]. Men are more frequently affected than women (Relative Risk (RR) = 1.3) and individuals of African American descent are at a higher risk in comparison to Caucasians (RR = 1.5) [3]. Despite some improvements in early diagnosis, surgical therapy, neoadjuvant therapy, adjuvant therapy and palliative interventions, the overall survival of patients with PC is still quite poor with only 6-9% of all patients being alive after 5 years (**Figure 4**) [6].

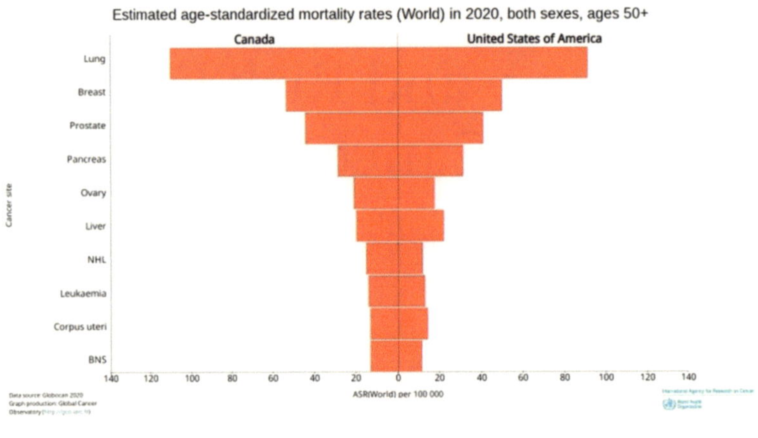

Figure 1.
Estimated age-standardized mortality rates of the most common types of malignancies in 2020 for patients older than 50 years in Canada and in the United States (data from the World Health Organization; https://gco.iarc.fr/).

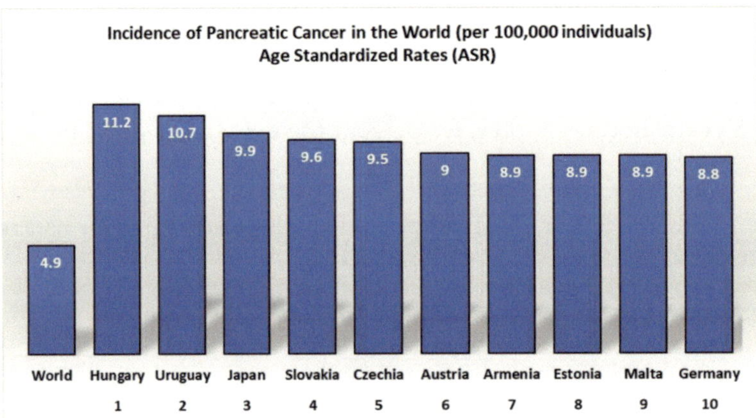

Figure 2.
Age-standardized incidence of pancreatic cancer in the world (4.9 per 100,000 individuals) and in selected countries with high incidence of the tumor (data from the World Health Organization; https://gco.iarc.fr/).

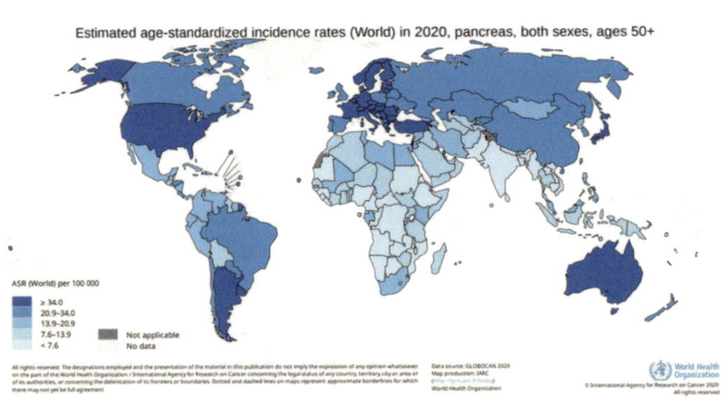

Figure 3.
Estimated age-standardized incidence of pancreatic cancer in the world for individuals older than 50 years (data from the World Health Organization; https://gco.iarc.fr/).

Type of cancer	Total number	Crude rate	ASR (World)	(%)
All cancers	18,094,716	232.1	190	100
Breast	2,261,419	58.5	47.8	12.5
Lung	2,206,771	28.3	22.4	12.2
Colorectum	1,931,590	24.8	19.5	10.7
Prostate	1,414,259	36	30.7	7.8
Stomach	1,089,103	14	11.1	6
Liver	905,677	11.6	9.5	5
Cervix uteri	604,127	15.6	13.3	3.3
Esophagus	604,100	7.8	6.3	3.3
Thyroid	586,202	7.5	6.6	3.2
Bladder	573,278	7.4	5.6	3.2
Non-Hodgkin lymphoma	544,352	7	5.8	3
Pancreas	495,773	6.4	4.9	2.7
Leukemia	474,519	6.1	5.4	2.6
Kidney	431,288	5.5	4.6	2.4
Corpus uteri	417,367	10.8	8.7	2.3
Lip and oral cavity	377,713	4.8	4.1	2.1
Melanoma of skin	324,635	4.2	3.4	1.8
Ovary	313,959	8.1	6.6	1.7
Brain and central nervous system	308,102	4	3.5	1.7
Larynx	184,615	2.4	2	1
Multiple myeloma	176,404	2.3	1.8	1
Nasopharynx	133,354	1.7	1.5	0.7
Gallbladder	115,949	1.5	1.2	0.6
Oropharynx	98,412	1.3	1.1	0.5
Hypopharynx	84,254	1.1	0.91	0.5
Hodgkin lymphoma	83,087	1.1	0.98	0.5
Testis	74,458	1.9	1.8	0.4
Salivary glands	53,583	0.69	0.57	0.3
Vulva	45,240	1.2	0.85	0.3
Penis	36,068	0.92	0.8	0.2
Kaposi sarcoma	34,270	0.44	0.39	0.2
Mesothelioma	30,870	0.4	0.3	0.2
Vagina	17,908	0.46	0.36	0.1

All ages, crude, and age-standardized rates per 100,000 individuals (data from the World Health Organization; https://gco.iarc.fr/).

Table 1.
Estimated number of patients diagnosed with cancer with exclusion of nonmelanoma skin cancer, worldwide in 2020.

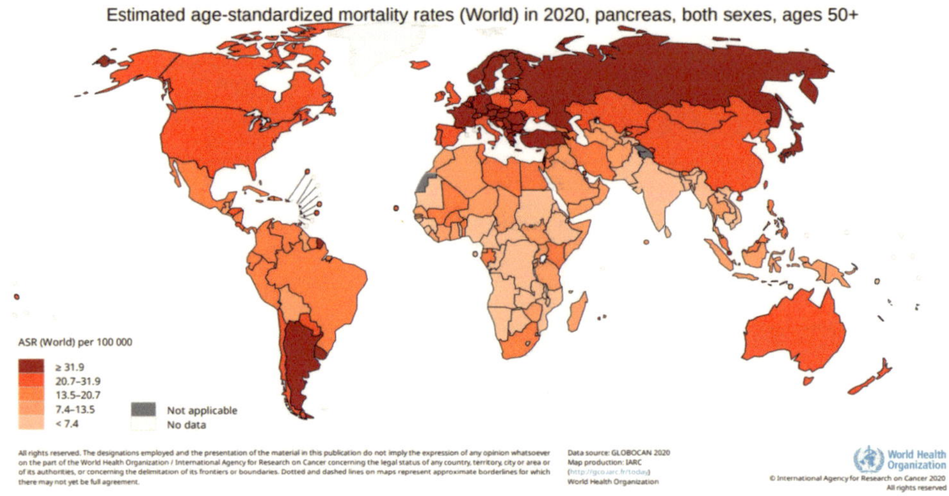

Figure 4.
Estimated age-standardized mortality rate of pancreatic cancer in different parts of the world for individuals older than 50 years (data from the World Health Organization; https://gco.iarc.fr/).

2. Risk factors

The strongest risk factor for PC is age. The incidence of PC increases significantly after the age of 50 and over 80% of PCs are diagnosed in patients older than 60 [7] (**Figure 5**).

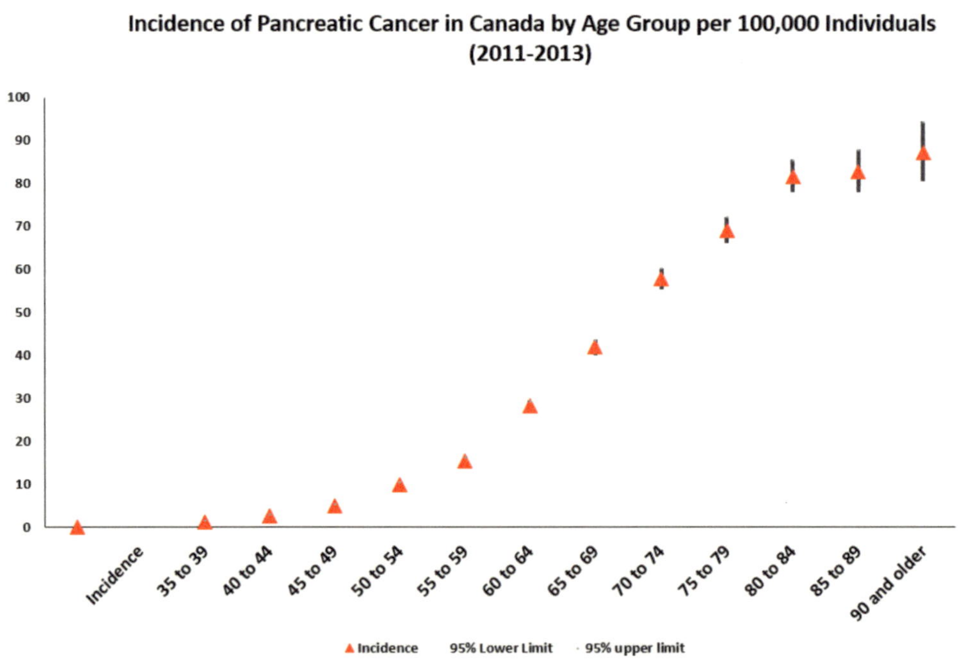

Figure 5.
Incidence of pancreatic cancer in Canada during the period between 2011 and 2013 per 100,000 individuals stratified by age.

2.1 Smoking

The risk of PC in smokers ranks second to lung cancer [8] and it is proportionate to the frequency (≥30 cigarettes per day: Odds Ratio (OR) = 1.75), duration (≥50 years: OR = 2.13), and cumulative smoking dose (≥40 pack/years: OR = 1.78) [9]. A meta-analysis of 82 studies from 4 continents has shown that cigarette smokers were diagnosed at significantly younger ages and had a 75% increased risk of developing PC in comparison to the regular population [10], and the risk persisted for 5 to 15 years after cessation [11]. In a case–control study of 808 PC patients matched against 808 healthy controls, in comparison to male counterparts, female smokers were at increased risk of developing PC as they suffered from a synergistic interaction between cigarette smoking, diabetes mellitus (OR = 9.3), and family history of PC (OR = 12.8) [12].

2.2 Diabetes

Nearly 80% of PC patients have either frank diabetes or impaired glucose tolerance at the time of their diagnosis [13]. Diabetes is often found concomitantly or during the two years preceding the diagnosis of PC [14]. Several studies have assessed the link between diabetes and PC with conflicting results. A meta-analysis of 11 cohort studies found that the relative risk for diabetic patients was 2.1 (95% CI 1.6–2.8) in comparison to nondiabetic individuals [15]. These findings were supported by another cohort study of 100,000 Danish diabetic patients that found a standardized incidence ratio of 2.1 (95% CI 1.9–2.4) [16]. A large prospective cohort study of 20,475 men and 15,183 women in the United States, has shown that the relative risk of dying from PC adjusted for age, race, history of cigarette smoking, and body mass index (BMI) was proportionate to the severity of diabetes. The RR was 1.65 for post-load plasma glucose levels between 6.7 and 8.8 mmol/L, 1.60 for levels between 8.9 and 11.0 mmol/L, and 2.15 for levels equal or more than 11.1 mmol/L [17]. Diabetes can present as an early manifestation of PC. Approximately 1% of new onset of diabetes in patients older than 50 is linked to PC [18]. Despite these findings, there is no evidence that screening patients for PC when newly diagnosed with diabetes [19] could reduce their mortality risk [5].

It is important to highlight that the link between abnormal glycemia and PC exists only for type II diabetes. A meta-analysis of 36 studies indicated that the OR of PC for patients with type II diabetes was 2.1 [20] while there are no reports showing an association between PC and type I diabetes [21].

Family history of diabetes does not appear to be a risk factor for PC [22]. On the other hand, a recent prospective study found that women with gestational diabetes are at a higher risk of developing PC with an estimated relative risk of 7.1 (95% CI = 2.8–18.0) [23]. Gapstur and colleagues [17] have proposed that high levels of insulin can cause abnormalities in the regulation of the insulin-like growth factor I (IGF1) receptor [19] that down-regulates the IGF binding protein 1, (IGFBP1) [20] causing an increase cell growth in PC cell lines [24, 25].

2.3 Alcohol

The role of alcohol in the predisposition of PC is controversial. Several studies have shown inconsistent findings due to multiple associations between alcohol consumption and other confounders such as cigarette smoking, lower socioeconomic status [26], and history of pancreatitis and diabetes [25]. A recent pooled analysis of 14 cohort studies with a sample of 862,664 individuals has shown a slight positive association between PC and alcohol consumption when larger than 30 gm/day (RR 1.22; 95% CI 1.03–1.45) [27]. On the other hand, a smaller epidemiological European study of 555 patients did not show any association between PC and alcohol consumption [28]. Yet, there is some evidence that compared with light drinkers, men consuming a large amount of hard liquor suffered from 62% increased risk of PC (95% CI 1.24–2.10) [11, 29] but this did not pan out for women and for beer and wine drinkers [29].

Although moderate alcohol consumption is not a risk factor, African Americans seem to be at a significantly higher risk of developing PC after adjusting for their drinking habits suggesting that racial differences play a role [30].

2.4 Pancreatitis

Several studies have shown a positive association between PC and history of pancreatitis. However, the magnitude of this phenomenon remains poorly understood [31, 32]. An international epidemiological study reported that both genders with chronic pancreatitis had an increased risk of developing PC independently from the cause of the disease [32]. A large case–control study indicated that chronic pancreatitis lasting more than 7 years was associated with a higher risk of PC (RR = 2.04; 95% CI 1.53–2.72) [33]. A large Italian study from 1983 to 1992 found similar results reporting that the risk increased after 5 or more years of chronic pancreatitis (RR in the first 4 years = 2.1, RR after 5 years = 6.9) [29]. These findings have been challenged by a more recent international study that showed that the risk was significantly increased only in the early years after the onset of pancreatitis. This observation suggested that pancreatitis might represent a manifestation of PC that becomes apparent only several years later rather than an independent risk factor for PC.

2.5 Hereditary pancreatitis

Hereditary pancreatitis affects 0.3 per 100,000 [34]. In 1996, it was found that hereditary pancreatitis was due to an autosomal dominant defect of the cationic trypsinogen gene (PRSS1) in 7q35 chromosome region [35]. Since then, more than 30 different PRSS1 mutations have been identified and reported in a few families. The risk of developing PC is particularly high for patients affected by hereditary pancreatitis who are at 53 times higher risk of developing the tumor in comparison to individuals without history of hereditary pancreatitis [36]. This observation was confirmed by another study that estimated a 40% cumulative risk of PC in patients with hereditary pancreatitis by the age of 70 [37]. For patients with paternal inheritance of hereditary pancreatitis, the cumulative risk of PC was even higher with a risk of up to 75% [37]. Patients with hereditary pancreatitis have high concentrations of cytokines, reactive oxygen molecules, and pro-inflammatory compounds that can lead to DNA damage, and despite DNA repair systems, these mechanisms seem responsible for the higher risk of genetic mutations leading to PC [33, 38].

2.6 Intraductal papillary mucinous neoplasms

The definition of intraductal papillary mucinous neoplasm (IPMN) is applied to a family of benign pancreatic cysts that can transform into PC [39]. The risk factors and the true incidence of IPMN are still unclear. These cysts produce mucin and are divided into two groups: IPMNs that affect the side branches of the pancreatic ducts and IPMN that affect the main pancreatic duct. Some patients have mixed IPMNs as they have cystic lesions in both the side branch and main pancreatic duct. IPMNs are responsible for 20–30% of PC cases. Current evidence suggests that only IPMNs affecting the main pancreatic duct are at high risk for malignant transformation. A recent meta-analysis [39] of 2411 patients with low-risk IPMNs and 825 patients with high-risk IPMNs has shown that the cumulative incidence of PC was significantly different between the two groups. For low-risk IPMNs, the cumulative incidence of PC was 0.02% at 1 year, 1.4% at 3 years, 3.1% at 5 years, and 7.7% at 10 years. On the other hand, for high-risk IPMNs, the cumulative incidence of PC was 1.9% at 1 year, 5.7% at 3 years, 9.7% at 5 years, and 24.6% at 10 years.

2.7 Genetic predisposition for pancreatic cancer

The presence of genetic predisposing factors for the development of PC has been an area of intense research during the last few decades. Case reports of families with multiple members diagnosed with PC suggest that for some patients, PC might be hereditary [40]. A large population study on twins identified hereditary factors for prostatic, breast, and colorectal cancers, however, this was not detected for PC [41]. A Canadian study on patients with suspected hereditary cancer syndromes found that the standardized incidence of PC was 4.5 (CI 0.54–16.) when cancer affected one 1st degree relative; the standardized incidence increased to 6.4 (CI 1.8–16.4) and 32 (CI 10.4–74.7) when two and three 1st degree relatives were affected, respectively [42]. This translates to an estimated incidence of PC of 41, 58, and 288 per 100,000 individuals, respectively, compared to 9 per 100,000 for the general population [43].

Brentnall et al. [44] and Meckler and colleagues [45] described examples of autosomal dominant PC in individuals presenting at early age (median age 43 years) and with high genetic penetrance (more than 80%). A mutation causing a proline (hydrophobic) to serine (hydrophilic) amino acid change (P239S) within a highly conserved region of the gene encoding paladin (PALLD) was found in all affected family members (family X). Another study has shown that the P239S mutation was only specific for the family X while it was not a common finding in other individuals with suspected familial PC [46]. Currently, genetic predisposition is thought to be responsible for 7–10% of all PC [47]. Genetic factors including germline mutations in p16/CDKN2A [48], BRCA2 [49–51], and STK 11 [52] genes are thought to increase the risk of PC. The combination of all these known genetic factors accounts for less than 20% of the familial aggregation of PC, suggesting that other genes play a role in the development of familial PC.

A systematic review and meta-analysis of studies on familial PC has shown that individuals with positive family history have nearly two-fold increased risk of developing PC (RR = 1.80, CI 1.48–2.12) [53]. Therefore, families with two or more cases may benefit from a comprehensive risk assessment involving collection of detailed family history information and data regarding other risk factors for PC [54]. A case–control study of PC in two Canadian provinces (Ontario and Quebec) assessed a total of 174 PC cases and 136 healthy controls. Information regarding the ages and sites of cancer was taken in 966 first-degree relatives of PC patients and for 903 first-degree relatives of the control group. PC was the only malignancy in excess in relatives of patients with PC, compared to the control group (RR = 5, p = 0.01). The lifetime risk of PC was 4.7% for the first-degree relatives and the risk was 7.2% for relatives of patients diagnosed before the age of 60 [55].

Besides the isolated aggregation of PC in some families, several other hereditary disorders predispose the development of PC in known familial cancer conditions [56].

These include hereditary pancreatitis, Peutz-Jeghers syndrome (STK11 mutation), familial atypical multiple mole melanoma (FAMMM mutation), familial breast cancer (BRCA1, BRCA2, PALB2, CDKN2A, ATM mutations) and ovarian cancer, Li-Fraumeni syndrome (TP53 mutation), Fanconi anemia, ataxia-telangiectasia, familial adenomatous polyposis, cystic fibrosis, and possible hereditary nonpolyposis colon cancer (HNPCC) or Lynch syndrome (MLH1, MSH2, MSH6, PMS2, EPCAM mutations) [4, 54, 57–59].

2.8 Familial pancreatic cancer registries

As the prognosis of PC is generally poor, there has been a strong interest to detect genes or other markers that could help identify high-risk patients in early stage. Although a precise genetic marker for this scope is not currently available, geneticists and epidemiologists have been profiling traits of high-risk families enrolled in registries established in North America and Europe [60]. Even if there is no standardized definition for familial PC, most authors apply the term to families with at least two first-degree relatives affected by PC in the absence of other predisposing familial conditions [60]. The creation of familial PC registries has been used not only for identification of genetic mutations but also for the screening of high-risk individuals. In selected centers in North America and Europe, screening programs for high-risk individuals have been implemented with the use of endoscopic ultrasound and computed tomography (CT) scan or magnetic resonance imaging (MRI). Such early diagnosis of PC within a comprehensive screening program is hoped to ultimately result in improved survival [61]. The discovery of the genetic bases of inherited PC continues to be an active area of research and in 2001 a multi-center linkage was formed to conduct studies aimed at the localization and identification of PC susceptibility genes (PACGENE) [62]. The complex nature of pedigree data makes it difficult to accurately assess risk based upon the simple counting of the number of affected family members, as it does not adjust for family size, age of onset of PC, and exact relationship between affected family members. Therefore, computer programs have been developed to integrate these complex risk factors and pedigree data. In April 2007 the 1st risk prediction tool for PC, PancPro (https://projects.iq.harvard.edu/bayesmendel/pancpro) was released [63]. This model provides accurate risk assessment for kindreds with familial PC as the receiver operating characteristic (ROC) curve was 0.75, which is considered good for predictive models.

3. Nutritional status

Several studies have explored the relationship between body mass index (BMI) lifestyle, diet, and the risk of PC, but uncertainty regarding the strength of this relationship still exists. A recent case–control study of 841 patients and 754 healthy controls showed that individuals with BMI of 25–29.9 had an OR of 1.67 (95% CI = 1.20–2.34) in comparison to obese patients (BMI of ≥30) who had an OR of 2.58 (95% CI = 1.70–3.90) independently of their diabetes status [64]. The duration of being overweight was significantly longer among patients with PC than among controls. Being obese or overweight, particularly in early adulthood, resulted in earlier onset of PC (age at presentation of PC was 61 years for overweight patients and 59 years for obese) when compared to the median age of diagnosis being 64 in the general population [65]. A few studies reported that central weight gain measured by

Age (more than 60 years)	
Smoking:	
Diabetes:	*Type II*
	Gestational diabetes
	Impaired glucose tolerance
Alcohol:	
Pancreatitis:	
	Acute
	Chronic
Genetic predisposition	
Family history:	
Hereditary disorders:	
	Hereditary pancreatitis
	Puetz-Jeghers syndrome
	FAMMM
	Familial breast and ovarian cancer
	Li-Fraumeni syndrome
	Fanconi anemia
	Ataxia-telengectasiatelangiectasia
	Familial adenomatous polyposis
	Cystic fibrosis
	HNPCC
	Lynch syndrome
Obesity:	
Intraductal Papillary Mucinous Neoplasms	

FAMMM: familial atypical multiple mole melanoma; HNPCC: hereditary nonpolyposis colon cancer.

Table 2.
Known risk factors for pancreatic cancer.

waist circumference and/or waist-to-hip ratio had a statistically significant increased risk compared to those with peripheral weight gain (RR = 1.45, 95% CI 1.02–2.07) [66, 67]. All the known risk factors for PC are summarized in **Table 2**.

4. Screening for pancreatic cancer

The role of screening for PC is not recommended for asymptomatic average-risk individuals [68, 69] as it is estimated that it would generate more harm than good. With an incidence of only 1.6% of individuals developing PC during their lifetime, Lucas et al. [68] estimated that even with an ideal screening tool with 99% sensitivity and 99% specificity, 1000 false positive results would be generated when the test is applied to 100,000 individuals. Current guidelines recommend that only healthy individuals with at least a 5% or higher risk of developing PC should be considered for screening programs [70] at age 50, or 10 years younger than the earliest diagnosis of PC in the family. These individuals must have two or more blood relatives diagnosed with PC with at least one affected first-degree relative [70, 71].

Guidelines also recommend that individuals with germline mutations in the genes listed above should consider screening beginning at age 50, or 10 years younger than the earliest pancreatic cancer diagnosis in the family, if they have a family history of PC. Some experts have recommended that all individuals with germline mutations in *STK11* (which causes Peutz-Jeghers syndrome) or *CDKN2A* (which causes familial atypical multiple mole melanoma [FAMMM] syndrome), ATM, BRCA1, BRCA2, CDKN2A, PALB2, PRSS1, STK11, TP53, and the Lynch syndrome mismatch repair genes undergo screening for PC regardless of their family history. Peutz-Jeghers syndrome patients are recommended to begin screening at ages 30 to 35. FAMMM syndrome patients are recommended to begin screening for PC at age 40. Magnetic resonance imaging (MRI) or endoscopic ultrasound (EUS) is the two radiological modalities recommended for the screening of patients considered at increased risk of developing PC.

5. Conclusions

PC is among the most common malignancies of the gastrointestinal system. Its incidence increases after the age of 50. Most patients diagnosed with PC have advanced disease at the time of their presentation. Age, cigarette smoking, alcohol abuse, chronic pancreatitis, and genetic factors are well-known predisposing factors for PC. Screening protocols for PC in the general population are not recommended as the incidence of PC is relatively low. The use of screening programs for high-risk patients is still under investigation.

Author details

Michele Molinari*, Hao Liu and Christof Kaltenmeier
Department of Surgery, University of Pittsburgh Medical Center, Pittsburgh, PA, United States

*Address all correspondence to: molinarim@upmc.edu

References

[1] International WCRF. Pancreatic Cancer Statistics. 2022. Available from: https://www.wcrf.org/cancer-trends/pancreatic-cancer-statistics/#:~:text=pancreatic%20cancer%20data-,Pancreatic%20cancer%20is%20the%2012th%20most%20common%20cancer%20worldwide.,most%20common%20cancer%20in%20women [Accessed: October 2, 2022]

[2] Jemal A, Siegel R, Ward E, Hao Y, Xu J, Thun MJ. Cancer statistics, 2009. CA: A Cancer Journal for Clinicians. 2009;**59**(4):225-249

[3] Shaib YH, Davila JA, El-Serag HB. The epidemiology of pancreatic cancer in the United States: Changes below the surface. Alimentary Pharmacology & Therapeutics. 2006;**24**(1):87-94

[4] Ghadirian P, Lynch HT, Krewski D. Epidemiology of pancreatic cancer: An overview. Cancer Detection and Prevention. 2003;**27**(2):87-93

[5] Lowenfels AB, Maisonneuve P. Epidemiology and risk factors for pancreatic cancer. Best Practice & Research. Clinical Gastroenterology. 2006;**20**(2):197-209

[6] Rawla P, Sunkara T, Gaduputi V. Epidemiology of pancreatic cancer: Global trends, etiology and risk factors. World Journal of Oncology. 2019;**10**(1):10-27

[7] Lin RT, Chen PL, Yang CY, Yeh CC, Lin CC, Huang WH, et al. Risk factors related to age at diagnosis of pancreatic cancer: A retrospective cohort pilot study. BMC Gastroenterology. 2022;**22**(1):243

[8] Neugut AI, Ahsan H, Robinson E. Pancreas cancer as a second primary malignancy. A population-based study. Cancer. 1995;**76**(4):589-592

[9] Lynch SM, Vrieling A, Lubin JH, Kraft P, Mendelsohn JB, Hartge P, et al. Cigarette smoking and pancreatic cancer: A pooled analysis from the pancreatic cancer cohort consortium. American Journal of Epidemiology. 2009;**170**(4):403-413

[10] Brand RE, Greer JB, Zolotarevsky E, Brand R, Du H, Simeone D, et al. Pancreatic cancer patients who smoke and drink are diagnosed at younger ages. Clinical Gastroenterology and Hepatology. 2009;**7**(9):1007-1012

[11] Iodice S, Gandini S, Maisonneuve P, Lowenfels AB. Tobacco and the risk of pancreatic cancer: A review and meta-analysis. Langenbeck's Archives of Surgery. 2008;**393**(4):535-545

[12] Hassan MM, Bondy ML, Wolff RA, Abbruzzese JL, Vauthey JN, Pisters PW, et al. Risk factors for pancreatic cancer: Case-control study. The American Journal of Gastroenterology. 2007;**102**(12):2696-2707

[13] Permert J, Ihse I, Jorfeldt L, von Schenck H, Arnqvist HJ, Larsson J. Pancreatic cancer is associated with impaired glucose metabolism. The European Journal of Surgery. 1993;**159**(2):101-107

[14] Gullo L, Pezzilli R, Morselli-Labate AM. Diabetes and the risk of pancreatic cancer. The New England Journal of Medicine. 1994;**331**(2):81-84

[15] Everhart J, Wright D. Diabetes mellitus as a risk factor for pancreatic cancer. A meta-analysis. JAMA. 1995;**273**(20):1605-1609

[16] Wideroff L, Gridley G, Mellemkjaer L, Chow WH, Linet M, Keehn S, et al. Cancer incidence in a population-based cohort of patients hospitalized with diabetes mellitus in Denmark. Journal of the National Cancer Institute. 1997;**89**(18):1360-1365

[17] Gapstur SM, Gann PH, Lowe W, Liu K, Colangelo L, Dyer A. Abnormal glucose metabolism and pancreatic cancer mortality. Journal of the American Medical Association. 2000;**283**(19):2552-2558

[18] Chari ST, Leibson CL, Rabe KG, Ransom J, de Andrade M, Petersen GM. Probability of pancreatic cancer following diabetes: A population-based study. Gastroenterology. 2005;**129**(2):504-511

[19] Ogawa Y, Tanaka M, Inoue K, Yamaguchi K, Chijiiwa K, Mizumoto K, et al. A prospective pancreatographic study of the prevalence of pancreatic carcinoma in patients with diabetes mellitus. Cancer. 2002;**94**(9):2344-2349

[20] Huxley R, Ansary-Moghaddam A, Berrington de Gonzalez A, Barzi F, Woodward M. Type-II diabetes and pancreatic cancer: A meta-analysis of 36 studies. British Journal of Cancer. 2005;**92**(11):2076-2083

[21] Yalniz M, Pour PM. Diabetes mellitus: A risk factor for pancreatic cancer? Langenbeck's Archives of Surgery. 2005;**390**(1):66-72

[22] Silverman DT, Schiffman M, Everhart J, Goldstein A, Lillemoe KD, Swanson GM, et al. Diabetes mellitus, other medical conditions and familial history of cancer as risk factors for pancreatic cancer. British Journal of Cancer. 1999;**80**(11):1830-1837

[23] Perrin MC, Terry MB, Kleinhaus K, Deutsch L, Yanetz R, Tiram E, et al. Gestational diabetes as a risk factor for pancreatic cancer: A prospective cohort study. BMC Medicine. 2007;**5**:25

[24] Fisher WE, Boros LG, Schirmer WJ. Insulin promotes pancreatic cancer: Evidence for endocrine influence on exocrine pancreatic tumors. The Journal of Surgical Research. 1996;**63**(1):310-313

[25] Lowenfels AB, Maisonneuve P, Cavallini G, Ammann RW, Lankisch PG, Andersen JR, et al. Pancreatitis and the risk of pancreatic cancer. International pancreatitis study group. The New England Journal of Medicine. 1993;**328**(20):1433-1437

[26] Jiao L, Silverman DT, Schairer C, Thiebaut AC, Hollenbeck AR, Leitzmann MF, et al. Alcohol use and risk of pancreatic cancer: The NIH-AARP diet and health study. American Journal of Epidemiology. 2009;**169**(9):1043-1051

[27] Genkinger JM, Spiegelman D, Anderson KE, Bergkvist L, Bernstein L, van den Brandt PA, et al. Alcohol intake and pancreatic cancer risk: A pooled analysis of fourteen cohort studies. Cancer Epidemiology, Biomarkers & Prevention. 2009;**18**(3):765-776

[28] Rohrmann S, Linseisen J, Vrieling A, Boffetta P, Stolzenberg-Solomon RZ, Lowenfels AB, et al. Ethanol intake and the risk of pancreatic cancer in the European prospective investigation into cancer and nutrition (EPIC). Cancer Causes & Control. 2009;**20**(5):785-794

[29] Fernandez E, La Vecchia C, Porta M, Negri E, d'Avanzo B, Boyle P. Pancreatitis and the risk of pancreatic cancer. Pancreas. 1995;**11**(2):185-189

[30] Silverman DT, Brown LM, Hoover RN, Schiffman M, Lillemoe KD, Schoenberg JB, et al. Alcohol and pancreatic cancer in blacks and whites

in the United States. Cancer Research. 1995;**55**(21):4899-4905

[31] Bansal P, Sonnenberg A. Pancreatitis is a risk factor for pancreatic cancer. Gastroenterology. 1995;**109**(1):247-251

[32] Karlson BM, Ekbom A, Josefsson S, McLaughlin JK, Fraumeni JF Jr, Nyren O. The risk of pancreatic cancer following pancreatitis: An association due to confounding? Gastroenterology. 1997;**113**(2):587-592

[33] Farrow B, Evers BM. Inflammation and the development of pancreatic cancer. Surgical Oncology. 2002;**10**(4):153-169

[34] Weiss FU. Pancreatic cancer risk in hereditary pancreatitis. Frontiers in Physiology. 2014;**5**:70

[35] Whitcomb DC, Gorry MC, Preston RA, Furey W, Sossenheimer MJ, Ulrich CD, et al. Hereditary pancreatitis is caused by a mutation in the cationic trypsinogen gene. Nature Genetics. 1996;**14**(2):141-145

[36] Whitcomb DC, Applebaum S, Martin SP. Hereditary pancreatitis and pancreatic carcinoma. Annals of the New York Academy of Sciences. 1999;**880**:201-209

[37] Lowenfels AB, Maisonneuve P, DiMagno EP, Elitsur Y, Gates LK Jr, Perrault J, et al. Hereditary pancreatitis and the risk of pancreatic cancer. International hereditary pancreatitis study group. Journal of the National Cancer Institute. 1997;**89**(6):442-446

[38] Hingorani SR, Wang LF, Multani AS, Combs C, Deramaudt TB, Hruban RH, et al. Trp53(R172H) and KraS(G12D) cooperate to promote chromosomal instability and widely metastatic pancreatic ductal adenocarcinoma in mice. Cancer Cell 2005;7(5):469-483.

[39] Choi SH, Park SH, Kim KW, Lee JY, Lee SS. Progression of Unresected Intraductal papillary mucinous neoplasms of the pancreas to cancer: A systematic review and meta-analysis. Clinical Gastroenterology and Hepatology. 2017;**15**(10):1509-20 e4

[40] Hruban RH, Petersen GM, Goggins M, Tersmette AC, Offerhaus GJ, Falatko F, et al. Familial pancreatic cancer. Annals of Oncology. 1999;**10**(Suppl. 4):69-73

[41] O'Brien JM. Environmental and heritable factors in the causation of cancer: Analyses of cohorts of twins from Sweden, Denmark, and Finland, by P. Lichtenstein, N.V. holm, P.K. Verkasalo, A. Iliadou, J. Kaprio, M. Koskenvuo, E. Pukkala, A. Skytthe, and K. Hemminki. N Engl J med 343:78-84, 2000. Survey of Ophthalmology. 2000;**45**(2):167-168

[42] Lilley M, Gilchrist D. The hereditary spectrum of pancreatic cancer: The Edmonton experience. Canadian Journal of Gastroenterology. 2004;**18**(1):17-21

[43] Klein AP, Brune KA, Petersen GM, Goggins M, Tersmette AC, Offerhaus GJ, et al. Prospective risk of pancreatic cancer in familial pancreatic cancer kindreds. Cancer Research. 2004;**64**(7):2634-2638

[44] Brentnall TA, Bronner MP, Byrd DR, Haggitt RC, Kimmey MB. Early diagnosis and treatment of pancreatic dysplasia in patients with a family history of pancreatic cancer. Annals of Internal Medicine. 1999;**131**(4):247-255

[45] Meckler KA, Brentnall TA, Haggitt RC, Crispin D, Byrd DR, Kimmey MB, et al. Familial fibrocystic pancreatic atrophy with endocrine cell hyperplasia and pancreatic carcinoma. The American Journal of Surgical Pathology. 2001;**25**(8):1047-1053

[46] Zogopoulos G, Rothenmund H, Eppel A, Ash C, Akbari MR, Hedley D, et al. The P239S palladin variant does not account for a significant fraction of hereditary or early onset pancreas cancer. Human Genetics. 2007;**121**(5):635-637

[47] Lynch HT, Fitzsimmons ML, Smyrk TC, Lanspa SJ, Watson P, McClellan J, et al. Familial pancreatic cancer: Clinicopathologic study of 18 nuclear families. The American Journal of Gastroenterology. 1990;**85**(1):54-60

[48] Goldstein AM, Fraser MC, Struewing JP, Hussussian CJ, Ranade K, Zametkin DP, et al. Increased risk of pancreatic cancer in melanoma-prone kindreds with p16INK4 mutations. The New England Journal of Medicine. 1995;**333**(15):970-974

[49] Goggins M, Schutte M, Lu J, Moskaluk CA, Weinstein CL, Petersen GM, et al. Germline BRCA2 gene mutations in patients with apparently sporadic pancreatic carcinomas. Cancer Research. 1996;**56**(23):5360-5364

[50] Hahn SA, Greenhalf B, Ellis I, Sina-Frey M, Rieder H, Korte B, et al. BRCA2 germline mutations in familial pancreatic carcinoma. Journal of the National Cancer Institute. 2003;**95**(3):214-221

[51] Murphy KM, Brune KA, Griffin C, Sollenberger JE, Petersen GM, Bansal R, et al. Evaluation of candidate genes MAP2K4, MADH4, ACVR1B, and BRCA2 in familial pancreatic cancer: Deleterious BRCA2 mutations in 17%. Cancer Research. 2002;**62**(13):3789-3793

[52] Su GH, Hruban RH, Bansal RK, Bova GS, Tang DJ, Shekher MC, et al. Germline and somatic mutations of the STK11/LKB1 Peutz-Jeghers gene in pancreatic and biliary cancers. The American Journal of Pathology. 1999;**154**(6):1835-1840

[53] Permuth-Wey J, Egan KM. Family history is a significant risk factor for pancreatic cancer: Results from a systematic review and meta-analysis. Familial Cancer. 2009;**8**(2):109-117

[54] Shi C, Hruban RH, Klein AP. Familial pancreatic cancer. Archives of Pathology & Laboratory Medicine. 2009;**133**(3):365-374

[55] Ghadirian P, Liu G, Gallinger S, Schmocker B, Paradis AJ, Lal G, et al. Risk of pancreatic cancer among individuals with a family history of cancer of the pancreas. International Journal of Cancer. 2002;**97**(6):807-810

[56] Bartsch DK, Kress R, Sina-Frey M, Grutzmann R, Gerdes B, Pilarsky C, et al. Prevalence of familial pancreatic cancer in Germany. International Journal of Cancer. 2004;**110**(6):902-906

[57] Bartsch DK. Familial pancreatic cancer. The British Journal of Surgery. 2003;**90**(4):386-387

[58] Landi S. Genetic predisposition and environmental risk factors to pancreatic cancer: A review of the literature. Mutation Research. 2009;**681**(2-3):299-307

[59] van der Heijden MS, Yeo CJ, Hruban RH, Kern SE. Fanconi anemia gene mutations in young-onset pancreatic cancer. Cancer Research. 2003;**63**(10):2585-2588

[60] Rieder H, Sina-Frey M, Ziegler A, Hahn SA, Przypadlo E, Kress R, et al. German national case collection of familial pancreatic cancer - clinical-genetic analysis of the first 21 families. Onkologie. 2002;**25**(3):262-266

[61] Hruban RH, Canto MI, Yeo CJ. Prevention of pancreatic cancer and strategies for management of familial pancreatic cancer. Digestive Diseases. 2001;**19**(1):76-84

[62] Petersen GM, de Andrade M, Goggins M, Hruban RH, Bondy M, Korczak JF, et al. Pancreatic cancer genetic epidemiology consortium. Cancer Epidemiology, Biomarkers & Prevention. 2006;**15**(4):704-710

[63] Wang W, Chen S, Brune KA, Hruban RH, Parmigiani G, Klein AP. PancPRO: Risk assessment for individuals with a family history of pancreatic cancer. Journal of Clinical Oncology. 2007;**25**(11):1417-1422

[64] Li D, Morris JS, Liu J, Hassan MM, Day RS, Bondy ML, et al. Body mass index and risk, age of onset, and survival in patients with pancreatic cancer. Journal of the American Medical Association. 2009;**301**(24):2553-2562

[65] Patel AV, Rodriguez C, Bernstein L, Chao A, Thun MJ, Calle EE. Obesity, recreational physical activity, and risk of pancreatic cancer in a large U.S. cohort. Cancer Epidemiology, Biomarkers & Prevention. 2005;**14**(2):459-466

[66] Larsson SC, Permert J, Hakansson N, Naslund I, Bergkvist L, Wolk A. Overall obesity, abdominal adiposity, diabetes and cigarette smoking in relation to the risk of pancreatic cancer in two Swedish population-based cohorts. British Journal of Cancer. 2005;**93**(11):1310-1315

[67] Berrington de Gonzalez A, Spencer EA, Bueno-de-Mesquita HB, Roddam A, Stolzenberg-Solomon R, Halkjaer J, et al. Anthropometry, physical activity, and the risk of pancreatic cancer in the European prospective investigation into cancer and nutrition. Cancer Epidemiology, Biomarkers & Prevention. 2006;**15**(5):879-885

[68] Lucas AL, Kastrinos F. Screening for pancreatic cancer. JAMA. 2019;**322**(5):407-408

[69] Tracer H, Sanou A. Screening for pancreatic cancer. American Family Physician. 2019;**100**(12):771-772

[70] Henrikson NB, Bowles EJA, Blasi PR, Morrison CC, Nguyen M, Pillarisetty VG, et al. Screening for pancreatic cancer: Updated evidence report and systematic review for the US preventive services task force. JAMA. 2019;**322**(5):445-454

[71] Canto MI, Harinck F, Hruban RH. International cancer of the pancreas screening (CAPS) consortium summit on the management of patients with increased risk for familial pancreatic cancer. Gut. 2014;**63**(1):178

Section 3

Cancer Pancreas: New Advances in Its Pathogenesis, Pathology and Management

Chapter 4

Pancreatic Cancer: Updates in Pathogenesis and Therapies

Emad Hamdy Gad

Abstract

Despite the progress in pancreatic cancer (PC) chemo/radiotherapies, immunotherapies, and novel targeted therapies and the improvement in its peri-operative management policies, it still has a dismal catastrophic prognosis due to delayed detection, early neural and vascular invasions, early micro-metastatic spread, tumour heterogeneities, drug resistance either intrinsic or acquired, unique desmoplastic stroma, and tumour microenvironment (TME). Understanding tumour pathogenesis at the detailed genetic/epigenetic/metabolic/molecular levels as well as studying the tumour risk factors and its known pre-cancerous lesions aggressively is required for getting a more successful therapy for this challenging tumour. For a better outcome of this catastrophic tumour, it should be diagnosed early and treated through multidisciplinary teams of surgeons, gastroenterologists/interventional upper endoscopists, medical/radiation oncologists, diagnostic/intervention radiologists, and pathologists at high-volume centres. Moreover, surgical resection with a negative margin (R0) is the only cure for it. In this chapter; we discuss the recently updated knowledge of PC pathogenesis, risk factors, and precancerous lesions as well as its different management tools (i.e. surgery, chemo/radiotherapies, immunotherapies, novel targeted therapies, local ablative therapies, etc.).

Keywords: cancer treatment, pancreas, pathogenesis, therapy, pathology

1. Introduction

Despite medical advances, pancreatic cancer (PC) is still a deadly challenging catastrophic tumour with a high mortality rate even after radical resection. It has a notable bad prognosis in comparison to the other malignant tumours due to its high malignant degree, gradual onset, typical symptoms defect, delayed discovery, difficult anatomical location, lower rate of curative resection, recurrence after resection, and high rate of chemo/radiotherapy resistance [1]. Globally; it is the 7th leading reason for cancer-related mortalities [2].

The most common cancer of the pancreas is pancreatic duct adenocarcinoma (PDAC) accounting for over 90% of cancers. Both the occurrence and progression of PDAC come from changes in some genes (i.e. KRAS oncogene mutational activation, inactivation of tumour suppressor genes (CDKN2A, TP53, and SMAD4), and/

or mutations in other genes involved in the cell cycle and apoptosis). Also, it occurs due to some risk factors (i.e. tobacco smoking, alcohol, obesity, diabetes, chronic pancreatitis, etc.) as well as some precancerous lesions (i.e. pancreatic intraepithelial neoplasia [PanIN], intra-ductal papillary mucinous neoplasm [IPMN], mucinous cystic neoplasms [MCN], etc.) [1].

Besides PDAC, there are some other pathological types of PCs (e.g. Acinar cell carcinoma, small cell carcinoma, cystadenocarcinomas, pancreatoblastoma, pancreatic neuroendocrine tumours [PNET], etc.) [1].

Depending on the tumour stage, resectable cancers are treated by surgical resection followed by adjuvant therapy. On the other hand, borderline resectable tumours are treated by neoadjuvant therapy followed by surgical resection. However, for patients with locally advanced or distant metastatic PCs, FOLFIRINOX (fluorouracil [5-FU], leucovorin, irinotecan, and oxaliplatin) and/or gemcitabine (a nucleotide analogue) plus albumin-bound paclitaxel (nab-paclitaxel) have been approved for use with high success [1, 3]. Lastly, future targeted therapies depending upon molecular pathways, tumour gene mutations and modulation of the tumour microenvironment (TME) are in progress under different phases of clinical trials [3].

2. Pathogenesis of PDAC

2.1 Genetics, molecular alterations, metabolic changes, and cancer pancreas

Understanding PDAC pathogenesis at the detailed genetic/epigenetic/metabolic/molecular levels as a tool to reach a more successful therapy for this challenging tumour remains an area of continuous aggressive research. The targeted molecular biology, whole exome sequencing studies, and genomic analyses showed that PDAC may occur due to mutational activation of some oncogenes/proto-oncogenes (i.e. KRAS, c-Myc, PAK4, MYB, HER2, etc.) and/or inactivation of some tumour suppressor genes (i.e. p16, TP53, SMAD4, CDKN2A, etc.), and/or mutations of DNA damage/repair (DDR) genes (i.e. ATM, BRCA1, BRCA2, PALB2, STK11, etc.), moreover, they can come from large chromosomal alterations (copy number alterations, chromosomal rearrangements, chromosomal instability from telomeres shortening, and clustered genomic rearrangements (chromothripsis)). Meanwhile; epigenetic DNA and histones alterations by methylation and acetylation respectively may be the leading causes of this catastrophic tumour [3].

The previous genetic alterations lead to changes in some signalling pathways (i.e. EGFR, TGFR, VEGF, IGF, Akt, NF-kB, Hedgehog, Wnt, Notch signalling, etc.) as well as other pathways (apoptosis and cell cycle pathways) causing PC progression [4]. So, those genetic alterations and changed signalling pathways became targets of the PC novel therapies (**Figure 1**).

MicroRNAs (miRNAs) are double-stranded small non-coding RNA molecules regulating gene expression at mRNA levels either by their degradation or translational inhibition. They have a role in PC initiation, pathogenesis, progression, proliferation, invasion, migration, and metastasis by affecting oncogenes (i.e. KRAS), tumour suppressor genes (i.e. P53), and/or signalling pathways (i.e. Notch) [5]. So they became a target for miRNAs-based novel therapies of PC in the preclinical levels (e.g. miRNAs natural modulating agents [i.e. curcumin], synthetic oligonucleotides that destroy oncogenic miRNAs and/or synthetic tumour suppressive miRNAs) [6].

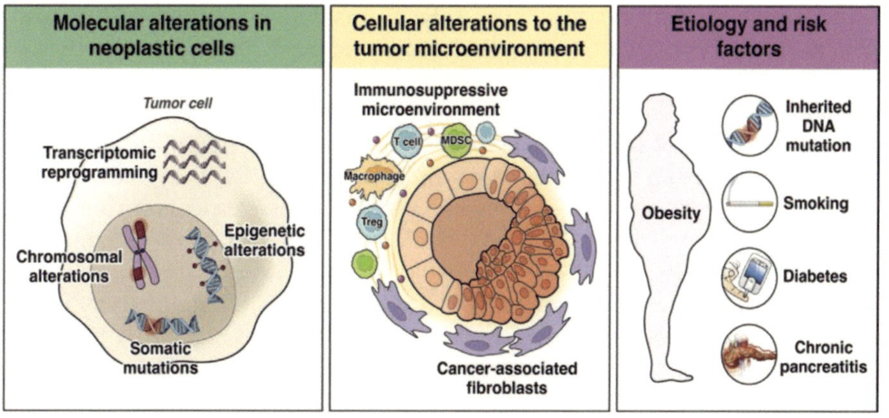

Figure 1.
Pathogenesis of PDAC. Taken from Wood et al. [3].

Long non-coding RNAs (lncRNA) such as HOTAIR are non-coding RNA molecules having lengths of more than 200 nucleotides with different cellular functions including transcriptional, post-transcriptional, and epigenetic regulation of gene expression. They have a critical role in PC progression by promoting proliferation, drug resistance, cell growth, migration, invasion, and metastasis. So, they will be a target for different therapies of PC soon [7].

Circular RNAs (CircRNAs) such as ciRS-7, circEIF6, etc. are single-stranded, non-coding covalently closed RNA molecules having a role in PC pathogenesis and progression by the followings: (1) Working as miRNAs decoys preventing them from binding to their target mRNAs leading to mRNAs stabilisation, perfect translation, and subsequently promoting tumour progression by proliferation, invasion, migration, metastasis, angiogenesis, augmenting chemotherapy resistance, and/or by inhibiting apoptosis. (2) Inhibiting post-translational modifications of proteins leads to protein stabilisation and tumour progression. (3) Acting as scaffolds for protein complexes leading to mRNA-protein complex formation enhancing mRNA expression and tumour progression. So, they will be a target for different therapies of PC soon (**Figure 2**) [7, 8].

Exosomes are small (30–100 nm) nano-scale extracellular vesicles with high stability, low immunogenicity, low cytotoxicity, and high membrane permeability

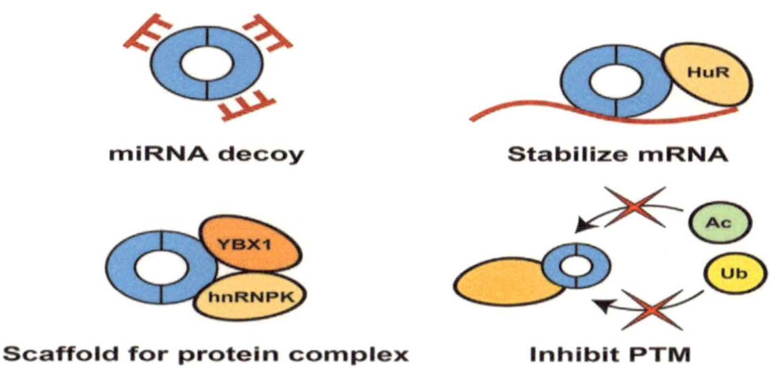

Figure 2.
Role of circRNAs in PC pathogenesis taken from Seimiya et al. [8].

containing cellular constituents (i.e. DNA, RNA, proteins, and lipids). They are secreted by all cell types into the circulation to transport biological components to other cells and tissues regulating intercellular communication. The exosomes originating from PC cells have a role in cancer growth, promotion, and metastasis through the induction of fibronectin secretion and the resulting inhibition of metastatic tumour infiltration by macrophages and neutrophils. So, they became a target for the future therapies of PC, also, they can act as vectors/carriers for therapeutics/ molecules transmission (drugs, miRNAs, circRNAs, lncRNA, small-interfering RNAs [siRNAs], etc.) [9–11].

By genomic (RNA-seq.) analysis, PDAC has been classified molecularly into the following four categories: (1) The squamous/quasi-mesenchymal/basal-like cancer; it is known by its high mesenchymal marker gene expression and by its worst prognosis when compared with the other categories, moreover, it is more sensitive to gemcitabine. (2) The pancreas progenitor/classical cancer is characterised by high epithelial marker gene expression and higher sensitivity to the EGFR inhibitors (erlotinib). (3) Immunogenic cancer is near to the pancreatic progenitor subtype but can be differentiated by the higher expression of the immune-related cell lines; furthermore, it has a higher sensitivity to immunotherapy, pembrolizumab. (4) The aberrantly differentiated endocrine-exocrine (ADEX)/exocrine-like cancer is characterised by a mixture of both endocrine and exocrine pancreatic cell lines [12–14].

PDAC may run in families (familial PC [families with at least two first-degree relatives with PDAC without observation of any other hereditary cancer syndromes]) and may be related to the following rare hereditary syndromes: (1) Hereditary pancreatitis with germ-line mutations in the cationic trypsinogen (PRSS1) gene, (2) Breast cancer susceptibility gene-1/2 (BRCA1/2) and PALB2 mutations, (3) Peutz–Jeghers syndrome due to mutations in the tumour suppressor gene STK11, (4) Familial atypical multiple-mole melanoma syndrome due to mutations in the tumour suppressor gene CDKN2A, (5) Hereditary non polyposis colon cancer (Lynch syndrome) due to mutation in mismatch repair (MMR) gene, (6) Familial adenomatous polyposis due to mutation of APC or MYTYH genes, (7) Ataxia telangiectasia due to mutation in the ataxia telangiectasia mutated (ATM) gene, (8) Li-Fraumeni syndrome Due to germ-line autosomal dominant mutation of TP53 gene, and (9) Werner's syndrome due to absence of WRN gene function [15–18].

2.2 The TME and its related factors in the pathogenesis of cancer pancreas

The PDAC TME is composed mainly of pancreatic stellate cells (PSC), immune cells, inflammatory cells, endothelial cells, extracellular matrix (ECM), neuronal cells. Also, soluble proteins like growth factors and cytokines have a main role in cancer pathogenesis, progression, and chemo-resistance through the followings: (1) The tumour has a dense desmoplastic stroma (comes mainly from PSC) with accumulation of a large amount of ECM (i.e. collagens, elastins, hyaluronan, etc.) leading to isolation of the tumour mass, severe hypoxia, and hypo-perfusion preventing drugs and immune cells from reaching the tumour cells; moreover activated PSCs promote cancer cell growth, proliferation, and invasion; (2) Immune cell changes (i.e. abundance of cells like myeloid-derived suppressor cells, tumour-associated macrophages (TAMs), and tumour-associated neutrophils and depletion of others like dendritic cells and anticancer T cells) promote immunosuppressive microenvironment preventing immune-mediated targeting of the tumour; (3) The cancer associated fibroblasts (CAF) have a role through metabolic support of the tumour, immune modulation of its microenvironment, promotion of cancer cell growth, survival, and invasion, and drug resistance; (4) Inflammatory process components (i.e. cytokines like TNF-α, IL-6, interferon-γ, and free radicals) have a role in PC promotion and progression. So, modulation of this TME became the target of many novel targeted therapies of PDAC in different recent clinical trials (**Figures 1** and **3**) [2, 3, 14, 19–23].

The developmental shift of PDAC cells from the epithelial to the mesenchymal or fibroblastoid phenotype epithelial mesenchymal transmission (EMT) is considered a vital step in the progression of the primary tumours to the invasive/metastatic/drug-resistant ones. It is a developmental process characterised by the degradation of the adherens and tight junctions of the epithelial cells to be converted to highly mobile and invasive mesenchymal cells. Molecularly, it is associated with decreasing levels of E-cadherin and conversely increasing levels of N-cadherin. In addition, it is associated with different signalling pathways of PC progression (i.e. Notch.), and with pancreatic cancer stem cell (PCSC) induction. This EMT enables cells to invade the surrounding tissues, the circulation, and finally to disseminate to distant sites [12, 24].

Due to their self-renewing and differentiation capabilities, PCSCs have a role in PC initiating and progression through tumour growth, invasion, metastasis, recurrence, and chemo/radio-resistance. They are regulated by different signalling pathways (i.e. Notch, Hedgehog, Wnt, etc.) and their chemo/radio-resistance comes from DNA repair capacity, increased DNA damage tolerance, tumour EMT, and higher levels of detoxification enzymes, epigenetic modifications, quiescence, and interaction with TME components. So, they became the target of many therapies of PC in the pre-clinical and clinical models [25].

The microbiota (i.e. bacteria, fungi, viruses, protozoa, etc.) normally inhabit human bodies mainly gastrointestinal tracts (GITs). They can be found also in oral cavities and different tissues like the pancreas playing an essential role in keeping body homeostasis; however; the microbiota imbalance (dysbiosis), and

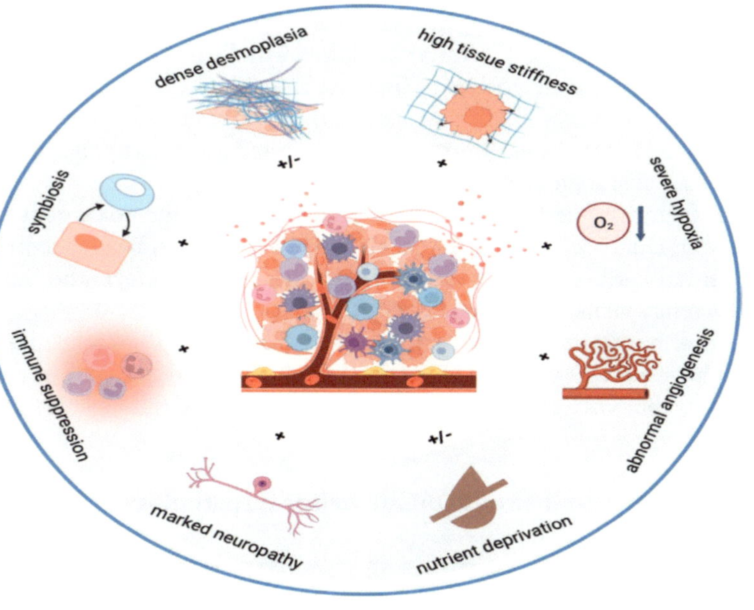

Figure 3.
The effect of PDAC TME on cancer pathogenesis and progression taken from Deng et al. [14].

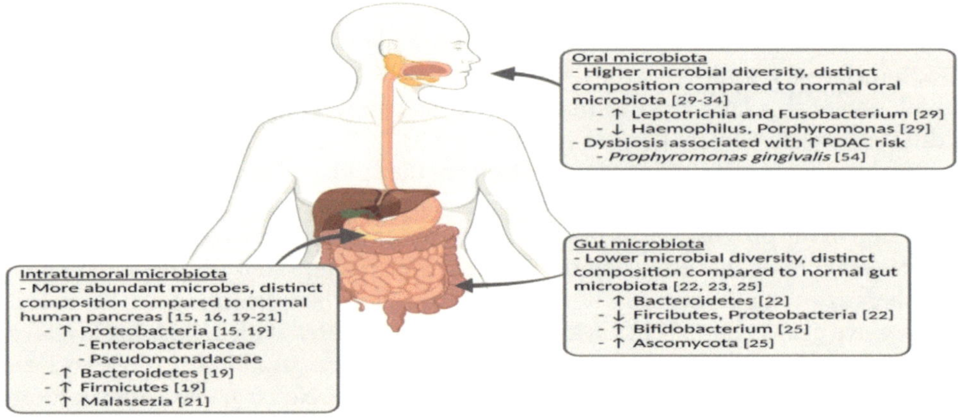

Figure 4.
Microbiota imbalance (dysbiosis) in PDAC; taken from Li et al. [26].

their combined genetic material (microbiome), have a major role in initiation and progression of tumours like PDAC by gene mutation, changing the TME immunity, altering tumour metabolism, promoting tumour inflammatory responses, and by promoting drug resistance (**Figure 4**). They can be detected by real-time quantitative polymerase chain reaction (qPCR) that can be confirmed by fluorescence in situ hybridization and immunohistochemistry and finally specified by amplified rRNA sequencing. Moreover, they became a target of novel therapies for PC in different clinical trials [26].

2.3 Risk factors of cancer pancreas

Several factors are increasing the risk of PDAC (**Figure 1**). One of these factors is cigarette smoking which promotes cancer development by DNA damage as well as by inflammation and fibrosis [27]. Similarly, diabetes mellitus either new-onset diabetes or long-standing one as well as obesity increase the risk of cancer pancreas through altered metabolic pathways, higher levels of adipocytokines, adrenomedullin, hyaluronan, vanin and matrix metalloproteinase, changed gut microbiota, increased PCSCs, increased EMT, and inflammation [9, 28].

The other factors related to PDAC occurrence are older age, male gender, processed meat, chemicals like asbestos, chronic pancreatitis, heavy alcohol consumption, and infections like hepatitis B virus, *Helicobacter pylori*, and human immunodeficiency virus infections [3, 29, 30].

On the other hand, patients with allergies (i.e. asthma, nasal allergies, hay fevers, etc.) have a lower risk of PC occurrence due to their active immune system [2]. Similarly, a diet with high fruit, vegetables, and folate reduces the risk of its occurrence [29].

2.4 The precancerous lesions of PDAC as well as its pathology

The invasive PDAC may arise from some curable resectable precancerous lesions; the most common of them is PanIN. These are less than 5 mm microscopic neoplasms involving the pancreatic ducts. However, a less common larger precancerous macro cystic lesion that involves the ducts and is also the IPMN [31]. Lastly, MCN is the

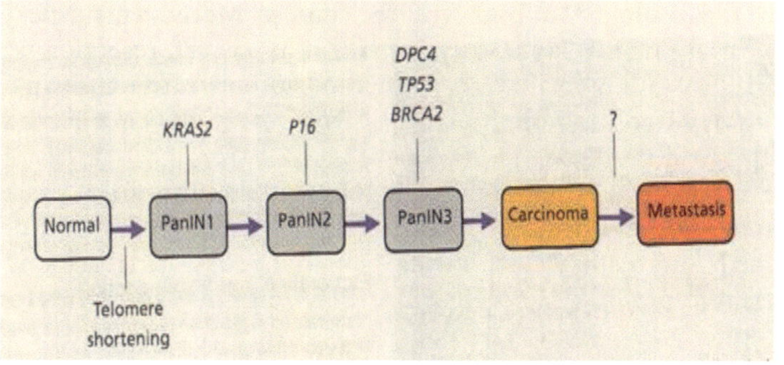

Figure 5.
Genetic progression of PanIN to invasive PDAC; taken from Kumari [16].

least common lesion. They do not involve the ductal system and have a characteristic ovarian-type stroma. They are more common in women and involve the pancreatic body and/or tail [32].

Morphologically, the previous precancerous lesions are sorted into low-grade and high-grade ones based on cytological and architectural atypia. The low-grade lesions have mild to moderate cytologic atypia and basally oriented nuclei. On the other hand, the high-grade ones have severe cytologic atypia, loss of nuclear polarity and marked architectural alterations [31, 33]. Regarding PanIN, their progression from normal epithelium to low-grade PanIN 1, 2 then to high-grade PanIN 3, and lastly to invasive PDAC is related to specific genetic alterations (i.e. early [KRAS mutation, telomere shortening], intermediate [p16/CDKN2A loss], and late [mutations of DPC4/SMAD4, TP53, BRCA2]). Moreover, the invasive PDAC is mostly associated with high-grade lesions (PanIN 3, and high-grade dysplasia of cystic lesions) (**Figure 5**) [16].

Regarding the pathology of PDACs, macroscopically, they are seen as fairly demarcated firm white-yellow masses with atrophic fibrotic neighbouring non-neoplastic pancreatic tissue; moreover, obstructive dilation of pancreatic ducts may be seen. On the other hand, the invasive tumour is characterised microscopically by mucin-producing glands elicited in a dense desmoplastic stroma with haphazard glandular arrangement, nuclear pleomorphism, glandular luminal necrosis, perineural, and lymphovascular invasions; moreover, they vary microscopically from well-differentiated duct forming carcinomas to poorly-differentiated carcinomas with glandular differentiation demonstrable only on immunolabelling [34, 35].

3. Treatment of PDAC

Despite the recent developments in diagnosis, surgery, radio/chemotherapy, immune therapy as well as targeted therapies of PDAC, it still has a very poor prognosis due to delayed detection, early micro-metastatic spread, drug resistance either intrinsic or acquired, unique desmoplastic stroma and TME, and tumour heterogeneities [36]. The 5-year survival rate after PC diagnosis may reach only 5–11%. However, for the very early diagnosed ones, it may rise to 85% and horribly; for the locally advanced or the metastatic ones, it may become less than 3% [1, 8, 16, 37]. For a better outcome of this catastrophic tumour, it should be diagnosed early and treated through multidisciplinary teams of surgeons, gastroenterologists/interventional upper endoscopists, medical/radiation oncologists, diagnostic/intervention radiologists, and pathologists at high-volume centres. Moreover, surgical resection with a negative margin (R0) is the only cure for it. However, resection is associated with high morbidity and mortality, so, meticulous preoperative assessment and preparation are required for better outcomes after resection (i.e. biliary drainage and nutritional support if required) [3, 29, 38–40].

Despite less than 20% of patients having resectable tumours at presentation [41], this aggressive tumour can be classified into resectable, borderline resectable, locally advanced, and distant metastatic. We will discuss the treatment options of those different types of PC as well as the different novel therapies for this catastrophic tumour.

3.1 The resectable tumour

The resectable tumour that lacks distant metastases, has no abnormal LNs away from the surgical basin and has no vascular invasion (No tumour–artery interface [celiac axis, superior mesenteric artery (SMA), or common hepatic artery (CHA)], >180-degree tumour–vein interface [superior mesenteric/portal veins (SMV/PV)]) is managed through surgical (open, laparoscopic, or robotic) removal of the affected pancreatic region (i.e. pancreaticoduodenectomy, distal pancreatectomy+splenectomy, and whole pancreatectomy+splenectomy for cancers of head, body/tail and whole gland respectively) as well as standard/extended lymphadenectomy (NB: ≤15 LNs should be excised) followed by adjuvant chemo/radiotherapy for improving long-term outcomes. However, neoadjuvant therapy before resection may be used in this group of patients especially patients with markedly elevated CA19-9, huge primary tumours and huge regional lymph nodes for assessing the benefit of surgery and for improving its outcome. Moreover, preoperative biliary drainage should be avoided in this group of patients due to its related drawbacks except in neoadjuvant therapy patients, as well as cholangitis and/or high bilirubin (>15 mg/dL) patients [3, 29, 38–40].

The previous management is prescribed with good patient performance status (PS) (based on Eastern Co-operative Oncology Group [ECOG]) with no major comorbidities; however, if the PS is poor, the patients with resectable non-operable PC are managed by single-agent chemotherapy (i.e. gemcitabine, 5-FU, etc.) or supportive symptomatic treatment [42].

3.2 The borderline resectable tumours

In patients with borderline resectable tumours (i.e. tumours that lack distant metastases, have no abnormal LNs away from the surgical basin, tumours with reconstructable invasion of SMV/PV or > 180-degree encasement of SMA); the treatment starts by the neoadjuvant chemo-radiation therapy aiming at downstaging of the tumour before resection and improving margin-negative resection rates, followed by surgical resection±intra-operative electron radiation therapy. In this category of patients, relief of biliary obstruction by plastic stenting before the neoadjuvant therapy should be done, furthermore, intraoperative venous reconstructions can be performed when needed with acceptable outcomes, and the adjuvant therapy can be given postoperatively. On the other hand, in patients with poor PS, the management will be palliative single-agent chemotherapy or supportive care [3, 29, 40, 43].

3.3 The surgical procedures

Classic pancreatoduodenectomy (PD), pylorus-preserving PD, radical PD, standard PD, extended PD, distal pancreatectomy, and total pancreatectomy are known procedures for resection of PDAC [43, 44].

Classic PD involves the excision of the pancreatic head, gallbladder, bile duct, duodenum, and gastric antrum [45]. A wide Kocher manoeuvre is performed, and the gastrocolic ligament is divided, the pancreatic neck is then dissected off the SMV. The porta hepatis dissection starts by exposing the CHA, and then identification and ligation of the gastroduodenal and right gastric arteries are performed. Then the PV is dissected off the pancreatic neck. Cholecystectomy as well as division of the common hepatic duct is then performed. The gastric antrum as well as the proximal 10 cm of jejunum is then resected. The pancreatic neck is then transected. Then the pancreatic head and uncinate process are dissected from the SMV/PV. (NB: some centres perform 'SMA-first' approaches to decrease blood loss and assess for R0 resection.) The soft tissue along the right lateral aspect of the SMA should be excised to prevent local recurrence. The resected specimen is removed as a single mass (en bloc resection) as shown in **Figure 6**. Then reconstruction starts with the pancreaticojejunostomy in the form of a retro colic end-to-side duct-to-mucosa anastomosis using interrupted sutures ± pancreatic stenting. Then, hepaticojejunostomy is performed distal to the previous anastomosis in a single layer of posterior continuous, and anterior interrupted sutures. Then finally, ante colic, end-to-side two layers gastrojejunostomy anastomosis is done around 50 cm from the hepaticojejunostomy anastomosis [43, 44].

In pylorus-preserving PD, the duodenum is divided distal to the pylorus taking care to preserve the gastroepiploic arcade. It maintains the integrity of the stomach and improves patients' quality of life. However, the radical PD operation is performed when there is no tissue plane between the tumour and SMV/PV by venous resection and reconstruction [43, 44].

In the PD procedure, the extent of the associated lymphadenectomy differs (standard vs. extended). In standard lymphadenectomy (standard PD), the resection involves gastric/pyloric nodes, anterior/posterior pancreaticoduodenal nodes, nodes to the right of the hepatoduodenal ligament/anterior to the CHA, and the ones to the right of the SMA. On the other hand, in extended lymphadenectomy (extended PD), the nodal excision includes nodes to the left/right of the hepatoduodenal ligament, common/proper hepatic arteries nodes, celiac axis nodes, all SMA nodes, and nodes in the anterolateral aspect of the aorta/the inferior vena cava. Moreover, the extended PD may be accompanied by the so-called total mesopancreas excision (TMPE) (i.e. a retropancreatic area,

(A) (B)

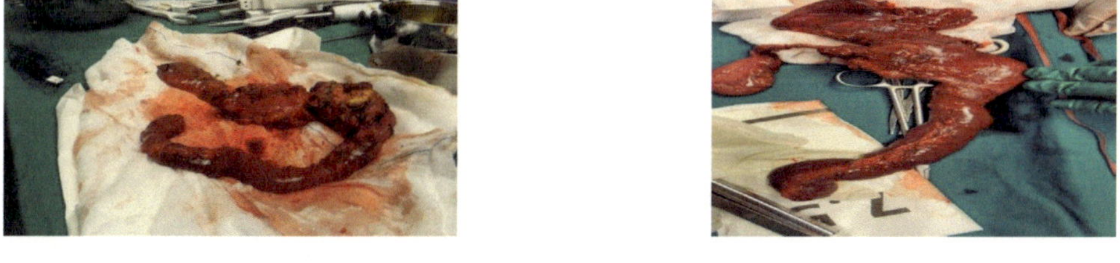

Figure 6.
A, B: Classic PD specimens (Author's operative work).

extending from pancreatic head, neck, and uncinated process to the aorto-caval groove, composed of loose areolar and adipose tissues, nerves, lymphatic as well as capillaries). The extended PD, radical PD, as well as TMPE, are all performed to reach R0 resection and to decrease recurrence [43, 44, 46]. Meanwhile, PD operations should be performed at high-volume centres (<10 surgeries/year) to get better survival due to experienced surgical/perioperative care at those high-volume centres [35, 47].

Distal pancreatectomy + splenectomy are performed for tumours of the pancreatic body/tail. The operation can be done through the left-to-right or right-to-left pancreatosplenectomy approaches with consideration of celiac axis nodal excision. However, total pancreatectomy is whole pancreas resection for tumours of the whole pancreas without liver or peritoneal metastases; it should be done in patients with strictly controlled clinical indications due to its multiple metabolic drawbacks [43, 44].

3.4 The neoadjuvant and adjuvant therapies

As mentioned before; neoadjuvant therapy is given to some patients with resectable tumours for chemosensitivity testing, better patient selection for surgery (no surgery if the disease progresses under neoadjuvant therapy), disease control, higher rate of R0 resection, tumour down-staging, post-surgical pancreatic leakage reduction, and improving postoperative survival outcomes. Also, it is given to borderline resectable cases for obtaining higher R0 resection rate, tumour down-sizing, and for improving post-resection survival rates [48]. Three to six cycles of neoadjuvant therapy can be given and the regimen differs according to the patient's PS, treatment response, etc. It may be FOLFIRINOX, gemcitabine plus nab-paclitaxel, 5-FU, gemcitabine, capecitabine, or combinations of the previous drugs± radiotherapy [39, 48].

On the other hand, six cycles of adjuvant therapy are recommended to be given within 4–12 weeks of surgery for decreasing postoperative recurrence and improving post-operative disease-free survival and overall survival rates. The proper regimen of adjuvant treatments varies according to many factors (i.e. patient's PS, treatment response, toxicities, etc.). FOLFIRINOX is the recommended adjuvant therapy in fit patients by various recent groups (i.e. European Society for Medical Oncology [ESMO], National Comprehensive Cancer Network [NCCN], and American Society of Clinical Oncology [ASCO] groups); however, drugs like gemcitabine plus nab-paclitaxel, 5-FU, gemcitabine, capecitabine, or combinations of them± radiotherapy can be given also [39, 48]. In addition, the radiotherapy may be in the form of photon radiotherapy or particle radiotherapy (proton or carbon ion radiotherapies); moreover, it can be given as external beam radiation therapy, brachytherapy, targeted three-dimensional conformal radiation therapy (3D-CRT), MR-guided radiotherapy and/or super gamma knife stereotactic conformal radiotherapy [3, 44].

3.5 E-the locally advanced/distant metastatic tumour

According to the recent European and American guidelines, the treatment of the locally advanced pancreatic cancer (LAPC) (i.e. non-reconstructable invasion of SMV/PV and/or < 180-degree encasement of SMA and/or tumour invading the first jejunal branch of the SMA without distant metastases) and the distant metastatic cancer is as follow: In patients with good PS, the first line treatment is FOLFIRINOX or gemcitabine plus nab-paclitaxel. However, the second line treatment is the alternative combination of the previous therapies (i.e. FOLFIRONOX treated patients are given gemcitabine plus nab-paclitaxel or gemcitabine (if nab-paclitaxel is not

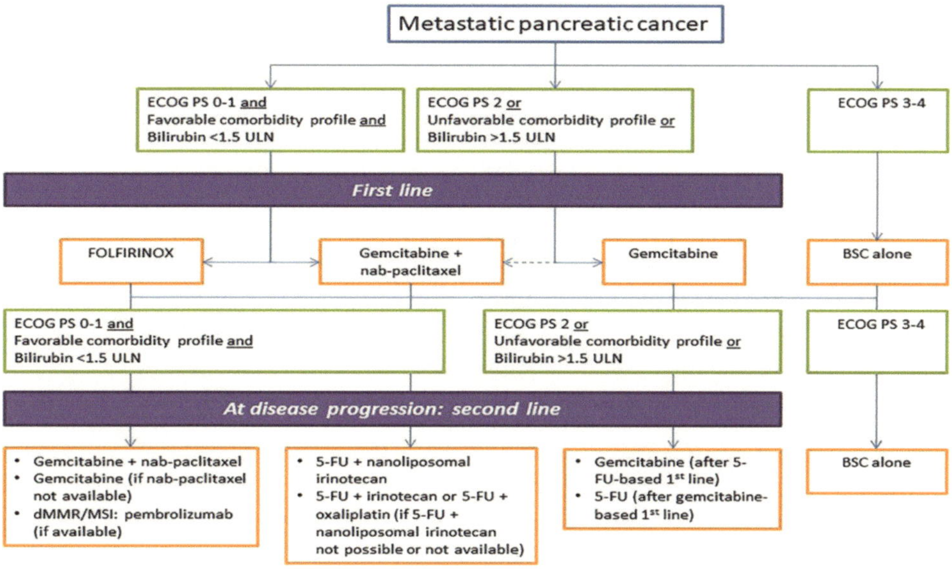

Figure 7.
Algorithm for first- and second-line chemotherapies in advanced PC; taken from Lambert et al. [48].

available) as a second line therapy while gemcitabine plus nab-paclitaxel treated patients take 5-FU+ nano liposomal irinotecan however, if nano liposomal irinotecan is not available, they take 5-FU+ irinotecan or 5-FU+ oxaliplatin as a second line) (**Figure 7**) [48]. The previous chemotherapeutics can be given as systemic IV therapy, and as transcatheter arterial infusion therapy; moreover, in the future, they can be given through exosomal transport or nanotechnology by combining them with nanoparticles (i.e. liposomes, micelles, iron nanoparticles, gold nanoparticle, etc.) [10, 36]. On the other hand, patients with poor PS are given single-agent chemotherapy (e.g. gemcitabine or 5-FU) or supportive symptomatic treatment (**Figure 7**) [3, 44, 48].

The previous palliative therapies of locally advanced/distant metastatic tumours should be combined with the following palliative therapies: (1) For biliary obstruction, surgical hepaticojejunostomy or endoscopic self-expanding metal stents are good options; (2) For gastric outlet obstruction, gastrojejunostomy and metal stenting are good options for patients with longer and shorter life expectancy respectively; (3) Intractable pancreatic pain is managed by percutaneous/endoscopic/surgical celiac plexus block; (4) Malnutrition can be managed by nutritional support. (NB: in some locally advanced non-metastatic cases, neoadjuvant therapy can be given then reassessment then curative surgery can be performed [conversion surgery]) [49].

Nanotechnologies are updated technologies developed to improve physicochemical properties (i.e. post administration solubility and circulation times) of the anticancer drugs (e.g. gemcitabine) to improve their efficacy and to decrease their resistance. Nanoparticles can act as PC drug carriers that increase drug absorption, permeability, circulation time, and tumour penetration. Also, they can decrease drug degradation, metabolism, and toxic side effects. They are promising future therapies for PC. Albumin-bound paclitaxel, liposomes, micelles, iron nanoparticles, and gold nanoparticles are examples of those nanoparticles [50, 51].

3.6 The loco-regional targeted therapies

The loco-regional targeted therapies performed either intraoperatively (open or laparoscopic), percutaneously, or as endoscopic ultrasound (EUS)-guided tools, have promising results in managing LAPC. These loco-regional therapies can be divided into thermal ablative therapies such as microwave ablation, radiofrequency ablation, cryo-ablation, and high intensity focused ultrasound ablative therapy, and non-thermal therapies like irreversible electroporation, and photodynamic therapies. Meanwhile, there are other EUS-guided therapies of LAPC such as radioactive seed implantation (brachytherapy; iodine-125), locally targeted radiotherapy, fine needle injection of chemotherapeutics (e.g. Gemcitabine, topical anti-KRAS therapy, etc.), biliary drainage (choledochoduodenostomy, hepaticogastrostomy, stenting, and gallbladder drainage), gastroenterostomy, celiac neurolysis, etc. [44, 52–55].

3.7 Updated novel therapies

Some novel therapies can be given to specific groups of patients. These are: (1) Patients with BRCA1/2 mutations are given platinum-based therapy or poly ADP-ribose polymerase (PARP) inhibitors (i.e. niraparib and olaparib); the drugs that promote cancer cell DNA damage or prevent its repair respectively causing cell cycle arrest and apoptosis [56]. Regarding platinum-based therapy, cisplatin has shown clinical benefits in different retrospective and prospective studies [3]. Moreover, Olaparib was approved by FDA in 2019 as a maintenance therapy for PC patients who responded to first-line cisplatin therapy as it increased their progression-free survival [56]. (2) PDAC with microsatellite instability (MSI)/MMR deficiency may respond to the immune therapy, pembrolizumab, which is an immune checkpoint inhibitor (anti-PD1 [programmed cell death protein-1]); it acts by preventing of binding of PD-1 to PD-L1 (programmed death ligand-1), this prevention leads to increased proliferation of the antitumour antigen-specific T cells as well as increased innate immunity to the tumour [3, 57]. Pembrolizumab is more effective in MSI-high tumours than MSI-low tumours, so it has been combined with chemotherapy, radio-therapy, and other immunotherapies in different clinical trials to increase its effect in MSI-low PDACs; an example of those trials is the COMBAT trial (NCT02826486) that concluded that the combination of pembrolizumab and CXCR4 antagonist with chemotherapy may improve tumour response to chemotherapy [3].

3.8 Immunotherapy under different phases of clinical trials (phases I, II, and III trials) with promising results that will have a main role in the future of PC therapy

(1) Immunotherapy targeting TME (i.e. Pegylated recombinant human hyaluronidase [PEG-PH20], in a phase Ib trial performed on stage IV PC patients, after they were given a combination of PEGPH20 and gemcitabine; the overall survival [OS] in high hyaluronic acid [HA] patients was higher than that in low HA patients) [58] (2) Immune checkpoint inhibitors like ipilimumab (immune checkpoint inhibitor, monoclonal antibody against CTLA-4, in a phase Ib trial when ipilimumab was given with GVAX [granulocyte macrophage colony-stimulating factor [GM-CSF vaccine]], the OS was longer than that observed when ipilimumab was given alone in advanced metastatic PC patients) [58]; moreover, there several ongoing clinical studies of Ipilimumab either as a monotherapy or as a combined medication with other immune checkpoint inhibitors, vaccines, chemotherapies, and/or tyrosine kinase inhibitors [59].

(3) Vaccines such as GVAX (it showed favourable results when given as combination therapy with different chemo-radiation therapies either in resectable or metastatic PCs in some clinical trials of phases I and II) [59]; mutant RAS peptide vaccine (in a Phase I/II study, the 10-year survival reached 20% after treatment with mutant RAS vaccine) [58]; Telomerase peptide vaccine (GV1001, despite showing promising results in a phase I/II trial of PC patients, it made no significant survival benefit when added to chemotherapy in other advanced PC phase III studies) [58, 59]; algenpantucel-L (an allogenic vaccine formed of αGal-expressing engineered PDAC cell lines; in a phase II study of PC patients, it showed promising results regarding disease-free survival [DFS] and OS when added to standard adjuvant chemotherapy) [59, 60]; K-Ras peptide vaccine (K-Ras mutated gene product; it showed promising results in phases I/II clinical trials when given alone or in combination with GVAX vaccine) [59]; Mucin-1 vaccine (it showed favourable outcomes in different phases I/II trials of PC patients) [59], VEGFR2 peptide vaccine (VEGFR2–169; it showed good results in a phase I trial of advanced PC when added to gemcitabine therapy) [59], Antigastrin vaccine (G17DT, it showed promising results when given either alone or in combination with other chemotherapies in different clinical trials of advanced PC populations) [59]; and lastly; dendritic cell (DC) vaccine (it showed acceptable results when given to PC patients in some trials) [59]. (4) Oncolytic viruses like ONYX-015 (adenovirus, in phase I/II trial of PC patients, its combination with gemcitabine was feasible and well-tolerated despite poor response) [58]; herpes simplex virus (HSV) (HF10, when it was given to six patients in a phase I trial, three were stable, one was in regression, and two were in progression) [58]; and Pelareorep (reovirus, it showed promising high viral replication in tumour cells and acceptable tolerance when combined with gemcitabine in a phase II study, also, it showed promising results and good safety when combined with chemotherapy and pembrolizumab in a phase Ib study) [60]. (5) Adoptive T-cell therapy (Chimeric antigen receptor [CAR]-T cell therapy, in phase I clinical study of patients with chemotherapy-refractory metastatic PC, the safety and efficacy of CAR-T- meso cells

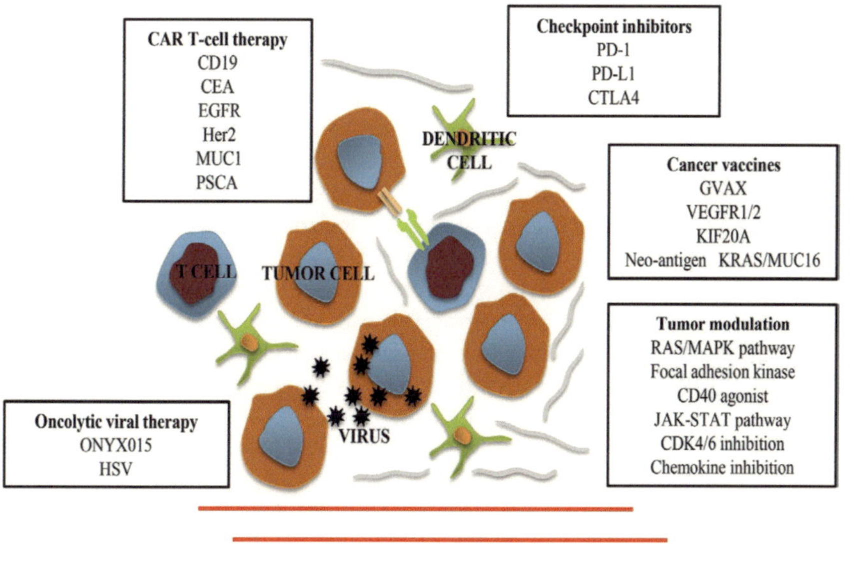

Figure 8.
Immunotherapy and PC; taken from Jiang et al. [58].

were promising) [58]. (6) Immunomodulatory agents like CD40 agonist antibodies (a tumour necrosis factor α receptor expressed on macrophages, B cells, and dendritic cells; in phase I clinical trial of advanced PC patients treated with both CD40 agonists and gemcitabine; the treatment was tolerable with promising results) [58]; JAK-STAT signalling pathway inhibitor (ruxolitinib, in phase II clinical trial of patients with metastatic PC who were treated with both ruxolitinib and capecitabine, the OS was significantly longer than that was observed in those patients treated with capecitabine alone) [58]; and CCR2 inhibitor (a chemokine receptor 2 inhibitors, PF-04136309, it showed favourable results when given with FOLFIRINOX in a phase Ib clinical trial of PC patients) [59]. 7-Monoclonal antibodies such as cetuximab (monoclonal antibodies against EGFR, when cetuximab was given with gemcitabine in a phase III study of the PC population; unfortunately, it did not show benefit) [61]; bevacizumab (monoclonal antibody against VEGFR, it also did not show benefit when combined with gemcitabine in a phase III study of PC patients) [61]; and MVT-5873 (monoclonal antibody against CA19.9, it showed promising results regarding safety, tolerability, and reduction of CA19.9 levels during the treatment course) [61] (**Figure 8**).

3.9 Other therapies that are probable promising future therapies

(1) Metabolic therapies like atorvastatin and metformin. (2) Antifibrotics like halofuginone. (3) Gene therapy like CYL-02. (4) Cell Cycle Check Point Inhibitors like abemaciclib and palbociclib. (5) Notch pathway inhibitor like Demcizumab. (6) Hedgehog signalling pathway inhibitor like vismodegib. (7) TGF-ß pathway inhibitor like trabedersen. (8) Therapeutic microbiota like MS-20. (9) M-TOR inhibitor like everolimus. (10) EGFR inhibitors (erlotinib). (11) Phytochemicals like curcumin. (12) Agents targeting KRAS mutant cancers like exosome-delivered KRAS siRNA (exosome) and anti-KRAS T cell transfer [12–14, 39, 49, 62, 63].

4. Conclusion

Despite the advance in the field of PC therapies (e.g. chemo/radio/immune/targeted therapies) and the well-developed peri-operative management policies for it during recent years, it still has a catastrophic poor prognosis due to its delayed detection, early neural/vascular invasions, early micro-metastatic spread, tumour heterogeneities, drug resistance either intrinsic or acquired, unique desmoplastic stroma and TME. It is fundamental to understand and make aggressive studies and researches about its pathogenesis at the different genetic/epigenetic/metabolic/molecular levels as well as to study its risk factors and its known precancerous lesions for getting a more successful therapy for it. Meanwhile, for reaching surgical R0 resection and a better outcome for this dismal challenging tumour, it should be diagnosed early and treated through multidisciplinary teams of surgeons, gastroenterologists/interventional upper endoscopists, medical/radiation oncologists, diagnostic/intervention radiologists, pathologists at high-volume centres.

Abbreviations

PDAC	pancreatic duct adenocarcinoma
PanIN	pancreatic intraepithelial neoplasia

IPMN	intra-ductal papillary mucinous neoplasm
MCN	mucinous cystic neoplasms
TME	tumour microenvironment
PC/s	pancreatic cancer/s
miRNAs	microRNAs
lncRNA	long non-coding RNAs
circRNAs	circular RNAs
siRNAs	small-interfering RNAs
BRCA	breast cancer susceptibility gene
MMR	mismatch repair gene
ATM	ataxia telangiectasia mutated gene
PSC	pancreatic stellate cells
ECM	extracellular matrix
TAMs	tumour-associated macrophages
CAF	cancer associated fibroblasts
EMT	epithelial to the mesenchymal
PCSC	pancreatic cancer stem cells
SMA	superior mesenteric artery
CHA	common hepatic artery
SMV/PV	superior mesenteric/portal veins
PS	performance status
ECOG	Eastern Co-operative Oncology Group
PD	pancreatoduodenectomy
SMV	superior mesenteric veins
PV	portal vein
TMPE	total mesopancreas excision
ESMO	European Society for Medical Oncology
NCCN	National Comprehensive Cancer Network
ASCO	American Society of Clinical Oncology
LAPC	locally advanced pancreatic cancer
EUS	endoscopic ultrasound
PARP	poly ADP-ribose polymerase
MSI	microsatellite instability

Author details

Emad Hamdy Gad
Hepatobiliary and Liver Transplantation Surgery Department, National Liver Institute, Menoufia University, Menoufia, Egypt

*Address all correspondence to: emadgadsalemaa@yahoo.com

References

[1] Chen H, Zhuo Q, Ye Z, Xu X, Ji S. Organoid model: A new hope for pancreatic cancer treatment? Biochimica Et Biophysica Acta. Reviews on Cancer. 2021;**1875**(1):188466. DOI: 10.1016/j.bbcan.2020.188466

[2] Afghani E, Klein AP. Pancreatic adenocarcinoma: Trends in epidemiology, risk factors, and outcomes. Hematology/Oncology Clinics of North America. 2022;**36**(5):879-895. DOI: 10.1016/j.hoc.2022.07.002

[3] Wood LD, Canto MI, Jaffee EM, Simeone DM. Pancreatic cancer: Pathogenesis, screening, diagnosis, and treatment. Gastroenterology. 2022;**163**(2):386-402.e1. DOI: 10.1053/j.gastro.2022.03.056

[4] Khan MA, Azim S, Zubair H, Bhardwaj A, Patel GK, Khushman M, et al. Molecular drivers of pancreatic cancer pathogenesis: Looking inward to move forward. International Journal of Molecular Sciences. 2017;**18**(4):779. DOI: 10.3390/ijms18040779

[5] Rachagani S, Macha MA, Heimann N, Seshacharyulu P, Haridas D, Chugh S, et al. Clinical implications of miRNAs in the pathogenesis, diagnosis and therapy of pancreatic cancer. Advanced Drug Delivery Reviews. 2015;**81**:16-33. DOI: 10.1016/j.addr.2014.10.020

[6] Li Y, Sarkar FH. MicroRNA targeted therapeutic approach for pancreatic cancer. International Journal of Biological Sciences. 2016;**12**(3):326-337. DOI: 10.7150/ijbs.15017

[7] Li Y, Al Hallak MN, Philip PA, Azmi AS, Mohammad RM. Non-coding RNAs in pancreatic cancer diagnostics and therapy: Focus on lncRNAs, circRNAs, and piRNAs. Cancers (Basel). 2021;**13**(16):4161. DOI: 10.3390/cancers13164161

[8] Seimiya T, Otsuka M, Fujishiro M. Roles of circular RNAs in the pathogenesis and treatment of pancreatic cancer. Frontiers in Cell and Development Biology. 2022;**10**:1023332. DOI: 10.3389/fcell.2022.1023332

[9] Pothuraju R, Rachagani S, Junker WM, Chaudhary S, Saraswathi V, Kaur S, et al. Pancreatic cancer associated with obesity and diabetes: An alternative approach for its targeting. Journal of Experimental & Clinical Cancer Research. 2018;**37**(1):319. DOI: 10.1186/s13046-018-0963-4

[10] Zhao X, Ren Y, Lu Z. Potential diagnostic and therapeutic roles of exosomes in pancreatic cancer. Biochimica Et Biophysica Acta. Reviews on Cancer. 2020;**1874**(2):188414. DOI: 10.1016/j.bbcan.2020.188414

[11] Hanjani NA, Esmaelizad N, Zanganeh S, Gharavi AT, Heidarizadeh P, Radfar M, et al. Emerging role of exosomes as biomarkers in cancer treatment and diagnosis. Critical Reviews in Oncology/Hematology. 2022;**169**:103565. DOI: 10.1016/j.critrevonc.2021.103565

[12] Grant TJ, Hua K, Singh A. Molecular pathogenesis of pancreatic cancer. Progress in Molecular Biology and Translational Science. 2016;**144**:241-275. DOI: 10.1016/bs.pmbts.2016.09.008

[13] Torres C, Grippo PJ. Pancreatic cancer subtypes: A roadmap for precision medicine. Annals of Medicine. 2018;**50**(4):277-287. DOI: 10.1080/07853890.2018.1453168

[14] Deng D, Patel R, Chiang CY, Hou P. Role of the tumor microenvironment in regulating pancreatic cancer therapy resistance. Cell. 2022;**11**(19):2952. DOI: 10.3390/cells11192952

[15] Rebours V, Boutron-Ruault MC, Schnee M, Férec C, Maire F, Hammel P, et al. Risk of pancreatic adenocarcinoma in patients with hereditary pancreatitis: A national exhaustive series. The American Journal of Gastroenterology. 2008;**103**(1):111-119. DOI: 10.1111/j.1572-0241.2007.01597.x

[16] Kumari LV. Pancreatic carcinoma: Review of literature. Journal of Evolution of Medical and Dental Sciences. 2015;**4**(37):6517-6531. DOI: 10.14260/jemds/2015/945

[17] Sawhney MS, Calderwood AH, Thosani NC, Rebbeck TR, Wani S, Canto MI, et al. ASGE guideline on screening for pancreatic cancer in individuals with genetic susceptibility: Summary and recommendations. Gastrointestinal Endoscopy. 2022;**95**(5):817-826. DOI: 10.1016/j.gie.2021.12.001

[18] Olakowski M, Bułdak Ł. Current status of inherited pancreatic cancer. Hereditary Cancer in Clinical Practice. 2022;**20**(1):26. DOI: 10.1186/s13053-022-00224-2

[19] Krishnamoorthy M, Lenehan JG, Burton JP, Maleki VS. Immunomodulation in pancreatic cancer. Cancers (Basel). 2020;**12**(11):3340. DOI: 10.3390/cancers12113340

[20] Khan AA, Liu X, Yan X, Tahir M, Ali S, Huang H. An overview of genetic mutations and epigenetic signatures in the course of pancreatic cancer progression. Cancer Metastasis Reviews. 2021;**40**(1):245-272. DOI: 10.1007/s10555-020-09952-0

[21] Beatty GL, Werba G, Lyssiotis CA, Simeone DM. The biological underpinnings of therapeutic resistance in pancreatic cancer. Genes & Development. 2021;**35**(13-14):940-962. DOI: 10.1101/gad.348523.121

[22] Capula M, Perán M, Xu G, Donati V, Yee D, Gregori A, et al. Role of drug catabolism, modulation of oncogenic signaling and tumor microenvironment in microbe-mediated pancreatic cancer chemoresistance. Drug Resistance Updates. 2022;**64**:100864. DOI: 10.1016/j.drup.2022.100864

[23] Sherman MH, Beatty GL. Tumor microenvironment in pancreatic cancer pathogenesis and therapeutic resistance. Annual Review of Pathology. 2023;**18**:123-148. DOI: 10.1146/annurev-pathmechdis-031621-024600

[24] Nattress CB, Halldén G. Advances in oncolytic adenovirus therapy for pancreatic cancer. Cancer Letters. 2018;**434**:56-69. DOI: 10.1016/j.canlet.2018.07.006

[25] Patil K, Khan FB, Akhtar S, Ahmad A, Uddin S. The plasticity of pancreatic cancer stem cells: Implications in therapeutic resistance. Cancer Metastasis Reviews. 2021;**40**(3):691-720. DOI: 10.1007/s10555-021-09979-x

[26] Li JJ, Zhu M, Kashyap PC, Chia N, Tran NH, McWilliams RR, et al. The role of microbiome in pancreatic cancer. Cancer Metastasis Reviews. 2021;**40**(3):777-789. DOI: 10.1007/s10555-021-09982-2

[27] Momi N, Kaur S, Ponnusamy MP, Kumar S, Wittel UA, Batra SK. Interplay between smoking-induced genotoxicity and altered signaling in pancreatic carcinogenesis. Carcinogenesis. 2012;**33**(9):1617-1628. DOI: 10.1093/carcin/bgs186

[28] Hassan MM, Bondy ML, Wolff RA, Abbruzzese JL, Vauthey JN, Pisters PW, et al. Risk factors for pancreatic cancer: Case-control study. The American Journal of Gastroenterology. 2007;**102**(12):2696-2707. DOI: 10.1111/j.1572-0241.2007.01510.x

[29] Ducreux M, Cuhna AS, Caramella C, Hollebecque A, Burtin P, Goéré D, et al. Cancer of the pancreas: ESMO clinical Practice guidelines for diagnosis, treatment and follow-up. Annals of Oncology. 2015;**26**(Suppl 5):v56-v68. DOI: 10.1093/annonc/mdv295

[30] Berrington de Gonzalez A, Sweetland S, Spencer E. A meta-analysis of obesity and the risk of pancreatic cancer. British Journal of Cancer. 2003;**89**(3):519-523. DOI: 10.1038/sj.bjc.6601140

[31] Basturk O, Hong SM, Wood LD, Adsay NV, Albores-Saavedra J, Biankin AV, et al. A revised classification system and recommendations from the Baltimore consensus meeting for neoplastic precursor lesions in the pancreas. The American Journal of Surgical Pathology. 2015;**39**(12):1730-1741. DOI: 10.1097/PAS.0000000000000533

[32] Zamboni G, Scarpa A, Bogina G, et al. Mucinous cystic tumors of the pancreas: Clinicopathological features, prognosis, and relationship to other mucinous cystic tumors. The American Journal of Surgical Pathology. 1999;**23**:410-422

[33] Matsuda Y, Furukawa T, Yachida S, Nishimura M, Seki A, Nonaka K, et al. The prevalence and Clinicopathological characteristics of high-grade pancreatic intraepithelial neoplasia: Autopsy study evaluating the entire pancreatic parenchyma. Pancreas. 2017;**46**(5):658-664. DOI: 10.1097/MPA.0000000000000786

[34] Rishi A, Goggins M, Wood LD, Hruban RH. Pathological and molecular evaluation of pancreatic neoplasms. Seminars in Oncology. 2015;**42**(1):28-39. DOI: 10.1053/j.seminoncol.2014.12.004

[35] Kamisawa T, Wood LD, Itoi T, Takaori K. Pancreatic cancer. Lancet. 2016;**388**(10039):73-85. DOI: 10.1016/S0140-6736(16)00141-0

[36] Tarannum M, Vivero-Escoto JL. Nanoparticle-based therapeutic strategies targeting major clinical challenges in pancreatic cancer treatment. Advanced Drug Delivery Reviews. 2022;**187**:114357. DOI: 10.1016/j.addr.2022.114357

[37] Badheeb M, Abdelrahim A, Esmail A, Umoru G, Abboud K, Al-Najjar E, et al. Pancreatic tumorigenesis: Precursors, genetic risk factors and screening. Current Oncology. 2022;**29**(11):8693-8719. DOI: 10.3390/curroncol29110686

[38] Silvestris N, Brunetti O, Bittoni A, Cataldo I, Corsi D, Crippa S, et al. Clinical Practice guidelines for diagnosis, treatment and follow-up of exocrine pancreatic ductal adenocarcinoma: Evidence evaluation and recommendations by the Italian Association of Medical Oncology (AIOM). Cancers (Basel). 2020;**12**(6):1681. DOI: 10.3390/cancers12061681

[39] Savani M, Shroff RT. Decision-making regarding perioperative therapy in individuals with localized pancreatic adenocarcinoma. Hematology/Oncology Clinics of North America. 2022;**36**(5):961-978. DOI: 10.1016/j.hoc.2022.07.003

[40] Matsuki R, Okano N, Hasui N, Kawaguchi S, Momose H, Kogure M, et al. Trends in the surgical treatment for pancreatic cancer in the last 30 years. Bioscience Trends. 2022;**16**(3):198-206. DOI: 10.5582/bst.2022.01250

[41] Zakaria H, Sallam AN, Ayoub II, Gad EH, Taha M, Roshdy MR, et al. Prognostic factors for long-term survival after pancreaticoduodenectomy for periampullary adenocarcinoma. A retrospective cohort study. Annals of Medicine and Surgery. 2020;**57**:321-327. DOI: 10.1016/j.amsu.2020.07.059

[42] Cui J, Jiao F, Li Q, Wang Z, Fu D, Liang J, et al. Chinese Society of Clinical Oncology (CSCO): Clinical guidelines for the diagnosis and treatment of pancreatic cancer. Journal of the National Cancer Center. 2022;**2**:205-215. DOI: doi.org/10.1016/j.jncc.2022.08.006

[43] Calvo FA, Asencio JM, Roeder F, Krempien R, Poortmans P, Hensley FW, et al. ESTRO IORT task force/ACROP recommendations for intraoperative radiation therapy in borderline-resected pancreatic cancer. Clinical and Translational Radiation Oncology. 2020;**23**:91-99. DOI: 10.1016/j.ctro.2020.05.005

[44] Li HY, Cui ZM, Chen J, Guo XZ, Li YY. Pancreatic cancer: Diagnosis and treatments. Tumour Biology. 2015;**36**(3):1375-1384. DOI: 10.1007/s13277-015-3223-7

[45] Rashad H, Abd El-Mabood EA, Elwan TH, Adbelmofeed AM, Salama RS, Gad EH. Reconstruction methods after pancreaticoduodenectomy for pancreatic carcinoma: Better method to prevent serious complications. The Egyptian Journal of Surgery. 2014;**33**:94-99. DOI: 10.4103/1110-1121.131662

[46] Xu J, Tian X, Chen Y, Ma Y, Liu C, Tian L, et al. Total mesopancreas excision for the treatment of pancreatic head cancer. Journal of Cancer. 2017;**8**(17):3575-3584. DOI: 10.7150/jca.21341

[47] Kommalapati A, Tella SH, Goyal G, Ma WW, Mahipal A. Contemporary Management of Localized Resectable Pancreatic Cancer. Cancers (Basel). 2018;**10**(1):24. DOI: 10.3390/cancers10010024

[48] Lambert A, Schwarz L, Borbath I, Henry A, Van Laethem JL, Malka D, et al. An update on treatment options for pancreatic adenocarcinoma. Therapeutic Advances in Medical Oncology. 2019;**11**:1758835919875568. DOI: 10.1177/1758835919875568

[49] Tempero MA, Malafa MP, Al-Hawary M, Behrman SW, Benson AB, Cardin DB, et al. Pancreatic adenocarcinoma, version 2.2021, NCCN clinical Practice guidelines in oncology. Journal of the National Comprehensive Cancer Network. 2021;**19**(4):439-457. DOI: 10.6004/jnccn.2021.0017

[50] Manzur A, Oluwasanmi A, Moss D, Curtis A, Hoskins C. Nanotechnologies in pancreatic cancer therapy. Pharmaceutics. 2017;**9**(4):39. DOI: 10.3390/pharmaceutics9040039

[51] Perko N, Mousa SA. Management of Pancreatic Cancer and its Microenvironment: Potential impact of Nano-targeting. Cancers (Basel). 2022;**14**(12):2879. DOI: 10.3390/cancers14122879

[52] Zhu J, Jin Z. Interventional therapy for pancreatic cancer. Gastrointestinal Tumors. 2016;**3**(2):81-89. DOI: 10.1159/000446800

[53] Linecker M, Pfammatter T, Kambakamba P, DeOliveira ML. Ablation strategies for locally advanced pancreatic cancer. Digestive Surgery. 2016;**33**(4):351-359. DOI: 10.1159/000445021

[54] Khokhar AS, Sher AF, Schattner M. Interventional endoscopy in the diagnosis and management of pancreatic adenocarcinoma. Chinese Clinical Oncology. 2017;**6**(6):63. DOI: 10.21037/cco.2017.12.02

[55] Narayanan G, Daye D, Wilson NM, Noman R, Mahendra AM, Doshi MH. Ablation in pancreatic cancer: Past, present and future. Cancers (Basel). 2021;**13**(11):2511. DOI: 10.3390/cancers13112511

[56] Perkhofer L, Gout J, Roger E, Kude de Almeida F, Baptista Simões C, Wiesmüller L, et al. DNA damage repair as a target in pancreatic cancer: State-of-the-art and future perspectives. Gut. 2021;**70**(3):606-617. DOI: 10.1136/gutjnl-2019-319984

[57] Wu J, Cai J. Dilemma and challenge of immunotherapy for pancreatic cancer. Digestive Diseases and Sciences. 2021;**66**(2):359-368. DOI: 10.1007/s10620-020-06183-9

[58] Jiang J, Zhou H, Ni C, Hu X, Mou Y, Huang D, et al. Immunotherapy in pancreatic cancer: New hope or mission impossible? Cancer Letters. 2019;**445**:57-64. DOI: 10.1016/j.canlet.2018.10.045

[59] Thind K, Padrnos LJ, Ramanathan RK, Borad MJ. Immunotherapy in pancreatic cancer treatment: A new frontier. Therapeutic Advances in Gastroenterology. 2017H;**10**(1):168-194. DOI: 10.1177/1756283X16667909

[60] Di Federico A, Mosca M, Pagani R, Carloni R, Frega G, De Giglio A, et al. Immunotherapy in pancreatic cancer: Why do we keep failing? A focus on tumor immune microenvironment, predictive biomarkers and treatment outcomes. Cancers (Basel). 2022;**14**(10):2429. DOI: 10.3390/cancers14102429 PMID: 35626033

[61] Chiaravalli M, Reni M, O'Reilly EM. Pancreatic ductal adenocarcinoma: State-of-the-art 2017 and new therapeutic strategies. Cancer Treatment Reviews. 2017;**60**:32-43. DOI: 10.1016/j.ctrv.2017.08.007

[62] Ducreux M, Seufferlein T, Van Laethem JL, Laurent-Puig P, Smolenschi C, Malka D, et al. Systemic treatment of pancreatic cancer revisited. Seminars in Oncology. 2019;**46**(1):28-38. DOI: 10.1053/j.seminoncol.2018.12.003

[63] Mohammed A, Janakiram NB, Pant S, Rao CV. Molecular targeted intervention for pancreatic cancer. Cancers (Basel). 2015;**7**(3):1499-1542. DOI: 10.3390/cancers7030850

Chapter 5

Pancreatic Tumorigenesis: Precursors, Genetic Risk Factors and Screening

Abdullah Esmail, Mohamed Badheeb and Maen Abdelrahim

Abstract

Pancreatic cancer (PC) is a highly fatal malignancy with a unique tumor microenvironment that limits the effectiveness of chemotherapeutics. PC develops from genetic mutations, cellular injury, and environmental exposure, progressing from precursor lesions to malignant neoplasms. This silent disease presents non-specific symptoms, including abdominal pain and painless jaundice. Serological and imaging evaluation aids in the diagnosis, with imaging modality selection dependent on cholestasis presence. The meticulous evaluation of vascular involvement and distant metastasis determines the tumor's resectability. Neoadjuvant therapy improves patient selection and limits micrometastases, while chemotherapy is the preferred treatment for unresectable cases. Early detection and personalized treatment are essential in improving PC's clinical outcomes.

Keywords: pancreatic cancer, tumorigenesis, screening, neoadjuvant therapy, pancreatic molecular profiling, pancreatic tumor microenvironment (TME)

1. Introduction

Pancreatic cancer (PC) is used interchangeably to describe pancreatic ductal adenocarcinoma, the most common pancreatic malignancy and one of the most fatal cancers worldwide [1, 2]. To gain a better understanding of PC pathogenesis, it is crucial to comprehend the pancreatic tumor microenvironment (TME). The TME is uniquely characterized by a dense desmoplastic fibrotic stroma in which extracellular matrix proteins (e.g., collagens), along with tumor-derived immune cells (e.g., neutrophils, macrophages), host immune cells (e.g., T-cells), fibroblasts, and activated pancreatic stellate cells (PSCs), form a dense barrier that limits the efficacy of different chemotherapeutics. This renders PC a difficult-to-treat illness [3–6]. Indeed, the tumorigenesis of PC involves genetic mutations, cellular injury, and environmental exposure that permit the transition into precursor lesions, which further progress into malignant neoplasms [7]. For instance, a constitutively active KRAS allows persistent downstream signaling with substantial cellular proliferation, resulting in ductal metaplasia [8, 9]. However, this process requires the acquisition of further genetic mutations, such as Angiopoietin-like 4, that permit the progression into pancreatic intraepithelial neoplasia

(PanINs) [10, 11]. Additionally, mutated TP53, CDKN2A, and SMAD4 accelerate PC growth and progression [12–15]. Moreover, various environmental factors are believed to contribute to PC tumorigenesis. Smoking has been shown to potentiate desmoplastic reactions by activating PSCs and the associated free radical injury [16]. Other contributing factors include obesity, primarily linked to its associated inflammatory status, which potentiates tumor progression [17, 18]. Furthermore, diabetes mellitus has been shown to over-activate PSCs, potentiating PC development [18]. Non-modifiable risk factors are also involved in PC development. Indeed, a higher incidence of PC was reported in patients of African American descent and patients with a family history of PC [19, 20]. Moreover, specific loci and familial cancer syndromes (e.g., hereditary non-polyposis colon cancer, familial atypical multiple mole melanoma syndromes) have been implicated in PC development [21]. Nonetheless, PC development is a multifactorial process, with various genetic and environmental factors contributing to its pathogenesis.

2. Clinical features of pancreatic cancer

The presentation of PC may vary based on the tumor location and stage. It is generally a silent disease, and if symptoms do occur, they tend to be non-specific, often leading to alternative diagnoses [22, 23]. Although "silent jaundice" is a classical symptom, abdominal pain is more frequently reported in 60–80% of cases [24, 25]. Tumors located in the head of the pancreas (70% of cases) tend to present with jaundice earlier in the course of the illness, while those in the body or tail present with jaundice later, indicating hepatic metastasis instead of biliary obstruction [26].

Syndrome	Associated features	Increased risk of PC	References
Hereditary non-polyposis colon cancer	Increase risk for endometrial, ovarian, gastric, colorectal, renal, gliomas, keratoacanthomas, and other malignancies	8.6-fold	[36]
Hereditary breast and ovarian cancer syndrome	Increased risk for breast (in males and females), ovarian, prostate, and skin (e.g., melanoma) malignancies	3–7%	[37]
Familial atypical multiple mole melanoma syndrome	Numerous atypical nevi resembling early melanoma, and a family history of melanoma Increase risk for lung, skin, larynx, and breast malignancies	13–22 folds	[38]
Familial adenomatous polyposis	Increased risk for desmoid tumors, gastric/duodenal, hepatoblastoma, and thyroid malignancies	4 folds	[39]
Peutz-Jeghers syndrome	Increased risk for colorectal, gastric, breast, ovarian, cervical, and testicular malignancies	15 folds	[40]
Li-Fraumeni syndrome	Increased risk for bone and soft tissue sarcomas and breast, brain, and adrenocortical malignancies	7 folds	[41]

Table 1.
Brief summary of familial cancer syndromes associated with pancreatic cancer (PC).

Other historical findings may include recent-onset diabetes, nausea or vomiting, anorexia, back pain, and weight loss.

In more advanced cases, pancreatic duct obstruction can result in symptoms of pancreatic failure, reported as post-prandial abdominal pain and steatorrhea. Fat malabsorption with associated vitamin deficiencies may also occur [24, 27–29]. Jaundice, hepatomegaly, and rarely epigastric mass may be noticed on examination [27]. Additionally, patients may experience recurrent venous stasis, resulting in splenomegaly with portal or splenic vein compression, ascites with inferior vena cava obstruction, and/or superficial thrombophlebitis (Trousseau's syndrome), palpable gallbladder (Courvoisier's sign), enlargement of the supraclavicular (Troisier's sign), or periumbilical (Sister Mary Joseph's node) lymph nodes may be observed [30–32]. Unfortunately, these findings are identified later in the course of the illness, indicating more advanced cases with poorer outcomes.

Clinicians should look for specific features of syndromes associated with PC, such as numerous atypical nevi in familial atypical multiple mole melanoma syndromes, mucocutaneous pigmentation in Peutz-Jeghers syndrome, and sebaceous tumors and cutaneous keratoacanthomas in patients with Lynch syndrome [33–35]. Syndromes associated with PC and their clinical features are summarized in **Table 1**.

3. Diagnosis of pancreatic cancer

The clinical presentation of PC is neither specific nor sensitive for establishing a diagnosis; therefore, suspected cases typically require serological and imaging testing. Liver function tests, including serum aminotransferase, bilirubin, and alkaline phosphatase, should be performed in all patients. The selection of subsequent testing primarily depends on the presence of jaundice or obstructive laboratory features (e.g., elevated direct bilirubin). In such cases, transabdominal ultrasound (TAUS) provides excellent sensitivity in detecting masses in the head of the pancreas and visualizing biliary tract patency or dilatation (**Figure 1**) [42, 43].

For anicteric patients who present with epigastric pain or other worrisome symptoms, such as weight loss, anorexia, or post-prandial flatulence, an abdominal computed tomography (CT) scan should be performed, which provides higher sensitivity in detecting lesions in the body and tail of the pancreas. In addition, a CT scan can be used initially, rather than TAUS, in cases of acute pancreatitis, as bowel gases may obscure the visualization of the biliary tract and the pancreas [44, 45]. If initial imaging is positive, further evaluation using a multi-phase contrast-enhanced, helical abdominal CT scan (i.e., pancreatic protocol) is the preferred option, accurate characterization of the pancreatic mass and resectability evaluation [46–48].

In cases where initial imaging (i.e., TAUS or CT scan) is negative, no further testing is required unless there is a strong suspicion that pancreatic cancer is the culprit of patient symptoms. In such cases, patients may undergo endoscopic retrograde cholangiopancreatography (ERCP), which allows for direct visualization of the biliary tract and pancreatic duct, tissue sampling for histopathological examination, and therapeutic decompression through stent insertion in selected cases. Alternatively, magnetic resonance cholangiopancreatography (MRCP) can be used in patients who are not qualified to undergo ERCP due to bowel obstruction or cases when ERCP fails to provide an informative visualization of the biliary tract [49–51]. When these modalities are negative, no further testing is required unless pancreatic cancer is

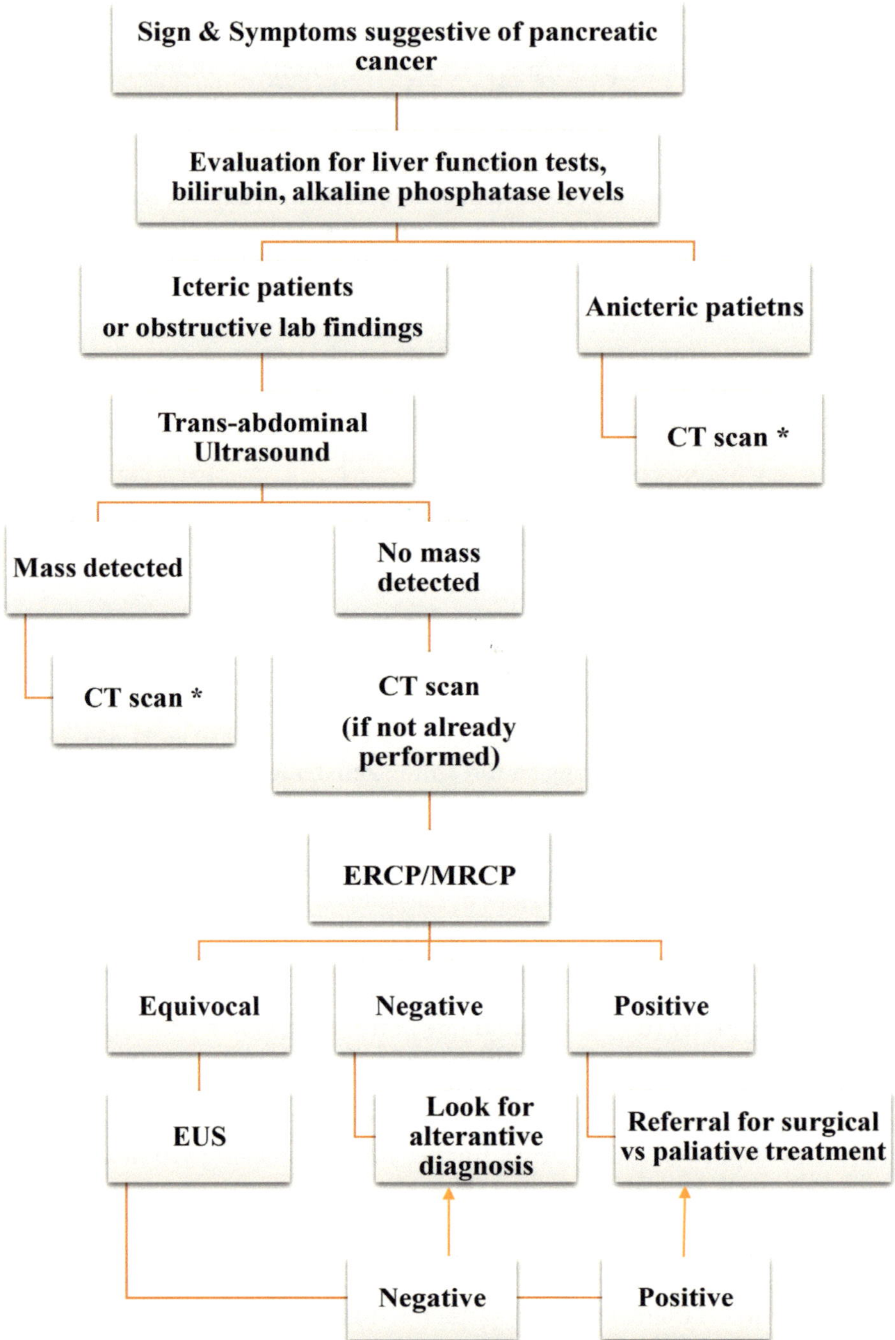

Figure 1.
*Simplified algorithm for pancreatic cancer diagnosis. * Pancreatic protocol to assess the resectability of the tumor.*

strongly suspected. In such cases, endoscopic ultrasound (EUS) may be sought to to assess further the presence of any pathologies, which should be sampled through fine needle aspiration (FNA). More recently, contrast-enhances EUS appeared to be a more feasible approach for tissue sampling in such cases [43, 52–54].

Tumor, node, metastasis (TNM) system by the American Joint Committee on Cancer manual is a widely-accepted staging system that aids in the assignment of patients based on the resectability of PC. Additionally, it provides prognostic information based on the stage; for instance, patients in stage Ia had an overall 5-years survival of 39% compared to 11% in stage III [48, 49]. Nevertheless, a four-grouped classification system is used by many clinicians, which classifies PC based on resectability into; resectable, borderline resectability, locally advanced, and metastatic PC [50]. Regardless of the system used, the ultimate goal is to determine the suitable patient for curative resection.

4. Screening of pancreatic cancer

Early diagnosis of PC has been shown to improve overall survival. Nevertheless, the low incidence of PC discourages the implementation of nationwide screening modalities due to the high risk of false positive cases that may undergo unnecessary invasive testing. Furthermore, there are currently no guidelines regarding the optimal screening for PC [55–58]. Therefore, patients should be selected cautiously and counseled regarding their risks, the benefits and harms of the test, and the probable outcomes of their testing.

Given the rarity of PC, a targeted screening approach may be the most suitable option. Initially, the identification of high-risk patients based on National Comprehensive Cancer Network (NCCN) recommendations [59] is primarily made on the basis of specific associated genetic mutations or syndromes to select the most appropriate age for screening initiation, as summarized in **Table 2**.

Various serological markers and liquid biopsies have been extensively studied; however, only Carbohydrate Antigen 19-9 (CA19-9) has gained approval from the Food and Drug Administration (FDA). Carcinoembryonic antigen (CEA), which is classically elevated in colorectal cancer, appears to have some diagnostic utility for detecting cancer but has lower specificity compared to CA19-9. The use of multiple biomarkers together provides higher cumulative sensitivity and specificity. For instance, CA19-9, CEA, CA125, and CA242 together had 90.4% and 93.8% sensitivity and specificity, respectively, substantially higher than any single marker [60–62]. More recently, liquid biopsies have gained tremendous interest as an alternative non-invasive method to detect PC. Mainly, circulating tumor DNA (ctDNA) and circulating tumor

Patient group	Age of initiation
High-risk genetic mutation, any of the: • ATM, BRCA1, BRCA2, MLH1, MSH2, MSH6, PALB2 or TP53 With a first-degree relative diagnosed with PC	Whichever earlier: • At 50 years old or • 10 years prior to the first PDAC in the family
Peutz-Jeghers syndrome	At 30–35 years old
Hereditary pancreatitis	• 40-years old or • 20 years following the onset of pancreatitis
CDKN2A mutation	• 40-years old or • Within 10 years of the first PDAC in the family

Table 2.
Screening age recommendations for high-risk patient groups.

Test	Sensitivity	Specificity	Advantage	Limitations
Serology				
CA19–9	80% [60]	75% [60]	Readily-available, FDA-approved	Low specificity, elevated in benign and non-PC cases, can be negative in up to 10% of Caucasians [66, 67]
CEA	45% [68]	89% [68]		Low sensitivity, elevated in benign and non-PC cases [68]
CA125	59% [69]	78% [69]	Not influenced by bilirubin levels, hence, its positive is the same in jaundiced and non-jaundiced individuals with PC [70]	Elevated in benign and non-PC cases [71]
CA242	66.2% [61]	80.14% [72]	May provide prognostic indications [73]	Ineffective early screening as a high level indicates a huge tumor burden [73]
IgG4	72% [74]	89% [74]		Limited usefulness to differentiate hereditary pancreatitis from PC [75]
Glycoproteomics	~90% [76]	90% [77]	Very high sensitivity and specificity can detect PC in its early stages	
Lipodomic profiling	>90% [78]	>90% [78]	Very high sensitivity and specificity may provide a prognostic indicator [78]	
Liquid biopsy				
CTCs and ctDNA	25–100% [63, 64]	95.4% [79]	May serve as recurrence, invasion, and metastasis predictors [63]	Variable sensitivity, and no standardized methodology to detect their recurrence [80]
cfDNA	76% [81]	59% [81]	Can detect genetic mutations (e.g., KRAS), and may serve as a recurrence, predictor [82, 83]	Low diagnostic accuracy, cannot detect the cancer cells origin [84]
Circulating miRNAs	92.5% [85]	90% [85]		The detection rate is tumor-burden dependent [86]
Circulating exosomes	75.4–100% [87]	92.6–100% [87]	High specificity can detect cancer DNA in its early stages [88]	

Table 3.
Different pancreatic cancer screening methods, their usefulness, and limitations.

cells (CTCs) are among the most promising. However, they are not readily available in many healthcare settings and have variable diagnostic accuracy [63–65]. **Table 3** summarizes different screening methods, their usefulness, and limitations.

Little is known regarding the best approach to screening for PC. Nevertheless, a comprehensive evaluation with cautious patient selection and integrative serological and imaging testing may be the most appropriate approach.

5. Management of pancreatic cancer

The management of PC is multidisciplinary. The tumor resectability should be evaluated initially with a multi-phase contrast-enhanced, helical chest and abdominopelvic CT scans. The tumor is considered resectable when confined to the pancreas with no metastasis or vascular encasement, such as the superior mesenteric artery/vein, celiac trunk, or common hepatic artery. Conversely, the presence of hepatic, peritoneal, or extra-abdominal metastasis renders the tumor unresectable [89, 90]. Nevertheless, in selective cases, the NCCN considers PC to be borderline unresectable. Examples of such cases include head of pancreas cancer that directly contacts the inferior vena cava, hepatic artery with no extension to the bifurcation, or tail/body PC with a celiac axis of 180 degrees or less [59]. For resectable PC that involves the head of the pancreas, the Whipple procedure is performed, including pancreatic head, duodenum, proximal jejunum, common bile duct, gall bladder, and a portion of the stomach resection (i.e., pancreaticoduodenectomy) [91, 92]. In contrast, distal pancreatectomy is typically performed in PC of the body/tail, which occasionally may include splenectomy [93]. Biliary drainage has been classically performed preoperatively in patients with obstructive jaundice. However, the clinical benefits of this approach are controversial; therefore, it should be reserved for patients with severe hyperbilirubinemia, protracted itching, or cholangitis [94–96].

Neoadjuvant therapy has been found to outperform initial surgical resection for PC in providing a more precise patient selection and possibly limiting micrometastases linked to PC recurrence even after surgical resection. In addition, lower margin-positive resections were observed with the use of neoadjuvant therapy [97–99]. However, there are currently no established guidelines regarding optimal chemotherapy. The FOLFIRINOX protocol and a combination of gemcitabine plus nab-paclitaxel have been used, but there is no sufficient evidence to support the superiority of each approach [100]. Thus, we recommend a multidisciplinary team evaluation that takes into account the patient's preferences, institutional experience, and cost-effectiveness when selecting the chemotherapeutic agents.

Metastatic and locally advanced PC are generally considered unresectable, and chemotherapy is the preferred approach for such cases. Although there is no consensus available for the preferred regimen, FOLFIRINOX or Gemcitabine-based protocols may be used. Different clinical trials have demonstrated the efficacy of each approach. However, FOLFIRINOX has shown a longer overall survival compared to Gemcitabine [101–105]. Patients who fail one protocol may be considered for the other after assessing their performance status. Additionally, patients should be re-evaluated for possible resection following chemotherapy, as tumor downstaging may permit resection.

List of abbreviation

CA19-9	carbohydrate antigen 19-9
CA125	cancer antigen 125

CA242	carbohydrate antigen 242
CEA	carcinoembryonic antigen
cfDNA	cell-free DNA
CT	computed tomography
ctDNA	circulating tumor DNA
CTCs	circulating tumor cells
ERCP	endoscopic retrograde cholangiopancreatography
EUS	endoscopic ultrasound
FDA	Food and Drug Administration
IgG4	immunoglobulin G4
MRCP	magnetic resonance cholangiopancreatography
NCCN	National Comprehensive Cancer Network
PanINs	pancreatic intraepithelial neoplasia
PC	pancreatic cancer
PSCs	pancreatic stellate cells
TAUS	transabdominal ultrasound
TME	tumor microenvironment
TNM	tumor, node, metastasis

Author details

Abdullah Esmail[1*], Mohamed Badheeb[2] and Maen Abdelrahim[1,3,4*]

1 Section of GI Oncology, Department of Medical Oncology, Houston Methodist Cancer Center, Houston, TX, USA

2 Internal Medicine Department, College of Medicine, Hadhramout University, Mukalla, Yemen

3 Weill Cornell Medical College, New York, NY, USA

4 Cockrell Center for Advanced Therapeutic Phase I Program, Houston Methodist Research Institute, Houston, TX, USA

*Address all correspondence to: aesmail@houstonmethodist.org and mabdelrahim@houstonmethodist.org

References

[1] Siegel RL, Miller KD, Fuchs HE, Jemal A. Cancer statistics, 2022. CA: A Cancer Journal for Clinicians. 2022;**72**(1):7-33

[2] Rawla P, Sunkara T, Gaduputi V. Epidemiology of pancreatic cancer: Global trends, etiology and risk factors. World Journal of Oncology. 2019;**10**(1):10-27

[3] DeClerck YA. Desmoplasia: A response or a niche? Cancer Discovery. 2012;**2**(9):772-774

[4] Hingorani SR, Petricoin EF, Maitra A, Rajapakse V, King C, Jacobetz MA, et al. Preinvasive and invasive ductal pancreatic cancer and its early detection in the mouse. Cancer Cell. 2003;**4**(6):437-450

[5] Cannon A, Thompson C, Hall BR, Jain M, Kumar S, Batra SK. Desmoplasia in pancreatic ductal adenocarcinoma: Insight into pathological function and therapeutic potential. Genes & Cancer. 2018;**9**(3-4):78-86

[6] Suklabaidya S, Dash P, Das B, Suresh V, Sasmal PK, Senapati S. Experimental models of pancreatic cancer desmoplasia. Laboratory Investigation; A Journal of Technical Methods and Pathology. 2018;**98**(1):27-40

[7] Petersen GM. Familial pancreatic adenocarcinoma. Hematology/ Oncology Clinics of North America. 2015;**29**(4):641-653

[8] Colicelli J, Human RAS. Superfamily Proteins and Related GTPases. 2004;**2004**(250) re13-re

[9] Hobbs GA, Der CJ, Rossman KL. RAS isoforms and mutations in cancer at a glance. Journal of Cell Science. 2016;**129**(7):1287-1292

[10] Basturk O, Hong SM, Wood LD, Adsay NV, Albores-Saavedra J, Biankin AV, et al. A revised classification system and recommendations from the Baltimore consensus meeting for neoplastic precursor lesions in the pancreas. The American Journal of Surgical Pathology. 2015;**39**(12):1730-1741

[11] Esposito I, Konukiewitz B, Schlitter AM, Klöppel G. Pathology of pancreatic ductal adenocarcinoma: Facts, challenges and future developments. World Journal of Gastroenterology. 2014;**20**(38):13833-13841

[12] Aguirre AJ, Bardeesy N, Sinha M, Lopez L, Tuveson DA, Horner J, et al. Activated Kras and Ink4a/Arf deficiency cooperate to produce metastatic pancreatic ductal adenocarcinoma. Genes & Development. 2003;**17**(24):3112-3126

[13] Jonckheere N, Vasseur R, Van Seuningen I. The cornerstone K-RAS mutation in pancreatic adenocarcinoma: From cell signaling network, target genes, biological processes to therapeutic targeting. Critical Reviews in Oncology/ Hematology. 2017;**111**:7-19

[14] Tang B, Li Y, Qi G, Yuan S, Wang Z, Yu S, et al. Clinicopathological significance of CDKN2A promoter hypermethylation frequency with pancreatic cancer. Scientific Reports. 2015;**5**:13563

[15] Sherr CJ. The INK4a/ARF network in tumour suppression. Nature Reviews Molecular Cell Biology. 2001;**2**(10):731-737

[16] Schaal C, Chellappan SP. Nicotine-mediated cell proliferation and tumor progression in smoking-related cancers. Molecular Cancer Research. 2014;**12**(1):14-23

[17] Rawla P, Thandra KC, Sunkara T. Pancreatic cancer and obesity: Epidemiology, mechanism, and preventive strategies. Clinical Journal of Gastroenterology. 2019;**12**(4):285-291

[18] Eibl G, Cruz-Monserrate Z, Korc M, Petrov MS, Goodarzi MO, Fisher WE, et al. Diabetes mellitus and obesity as risk factors for pancreatic cancer. Journal of the Academy of Nutrition and Dietetics. 2018;**118**(4):555-567

[19] Yadav D, Lowenfels AB. The epidemiology of pancreatitis and pancreatic cancer. Gastroenterology. 2013;**144**(6):1252-1261

[20] Arnold LD, Patel AV, Yan Y, Jacobs EJ, Thun MJ, Calle EE, et al. Are racial disparities in pancreatic cancer explained by smoking and overweight/obesity? Cancer Epidemiology, Biomarkers & Prevention. 2009;**18**(9):2397-2405

[21] Badheeb M, Abdelrahim A, Esmail A, Umoru G, Abboud K, Al-Najjar E, et al. Pancreatic tumorigenesis: Precursors, genetic risk factors and screening. Current Oncology (Toronto, Ont). 2022;**29**(11):8693-8719

[22] Macdonald S, Macleod U, Campbell NC, Weller D, Mitchell E. Systematic review of factors influencing patient and practitioner delay in diagnosis of upper gastrointestinal cancer. British Journal of Cancer. 2006;**94**(9):1272-1280

[23] Walter FM, Mills K, Mendonça SC, Abel GA, Basu B, Carroll N, et al. Symptoms and patient factors associated with diagnostic intervals for pancreatic cancer (SYMPTOM pancreatic study): A prospective cohort study. The Lancet Gastroenterology & Hepatology. 2016;**1**(4):298-306

[24] Schmidt-Hansen M, Berendse S, Hamilton W. Symptoms of pancreatic cancer in primary care: A systematic review. Pancreas. 2016;**45**(6):814-818

[25] Furukawa H, Okada S, Saisho H, Ariyama J, Karasawa E, Nakaizumi A, et al. Clinicopathologic features of small pancreatic adenocarcinoma. A collective study. Cancer. 1996;**78**(5):986-990

[26] Kalser MH, Barkin J, MacIntyre JM. Pancreatic cancer. Assessment of prognosis by clinical presentation. Cancer. 1985;**56**(2):397-402

[27] Porta M, Fabregat X, Malats N, Guarner L, Carrato A, de Miguel A, et al. Exocrine pancreatic cancer: Symptoms at presentation and their relation to tumour site and stage. Clinical & Translational Oncology: Official Publication of the Federation of Spanish Oncology Societies and of the National Cancer Institute of Mexico. 2005;**7**(5):189-197

[28] Holly EA, Chaliha I, Bracci PM, Gautam M. Signs and symptoms of pancreatic cancer: A population-based case-control study in the San Francisco Bay area. Clinical Gastroenterology and Hepatology: The Official Clinical Practice Journal of the American Gastroenterological Association. 2004;**2**(6):510-517

[29] Chari ST, Leibson CL, Rabe KG, Ransom J, de Andrade M, Petersen GM. Probability of pancreatic cancer following diabetes: A population-based study. Gastroenterology. 2005;**129**(2):504-511

[30] DiMagno EP. Pancreatic cancer: Clinical presentation, pitfalls and early

clues. Annals of Oncology: Official Journal of the European Society for Medical Oncology. 1999;**10**(Suppl 4):140-142

[31] Takhar AS, Palaniappan P, Dhingsa R, Lobo DN. Recent developments in diagnosis of pancreatic cancer. BMJ (Clinical Research ed). 2004;**329**(7467):668-673

[32] Khorana AA, Fine RL. Pancreatic cancer and thromboembolic disease. The Lancet Oncology. 2004;**5**(11):655-663

[33] Utsunomiya J, Gocho H, Miyanaga T, Hamaguchi E, Kashimure A. Peutz-Jeghers syndrome: Its natural course and management. The Johns Hopkins Medical Journal. 1975;**136**(2):71-82

[34] Eckerle Mize D, Bishop M, Resse E, Sluzevich J. Familial atypical multiple mole melanoma syndrome. In: Riegert-Johnson DL, Boardman LA, Hefferon T, Roberts M, editors. Cancer Syndromes. Bethesda (MD): National Center for Biotechnology Information (US) Copyright © 2009, Douglas L Riegert-Johnson; 2009

[35] Coquillard C, Boustany A, DeCoster RC, Vasconez HC. Muir-Torre syndrome presenting as a sebaceous carcinoma of the nasal ala. The American Surgeon. 2019;**85**(3):e115-e1e7

[36] Hoskins JW, Ibrahim A, Emmanuel MA, Manmiller SM, Wu Y, O'Neill M, et al. Functional characterization of a chr13q22.1 pancreatic cancer risk locus reveals long-range interaction and allele-specific effects on DIS3 expression. Human Molecular Genetics. 2016;**25**(21):4726-4738

[37] Petrucelli N, Daly MB, Pal T. BRCA1- and BRCA2-associated hereditary breast and ovarian cancer. In: Adam MP, Everman DB, Mirzaa GM, Pagon RA, Wallace SE, LJH B, et al., editors. GeneReviews(®). Seattle (WA): University of Washington, Seattle Copyright © 1993-2023, University of Washington, Seattle. GeneReviews is a registered trademark of the University of Washington, Seattle. All rights reserved; 1993

[38] Riker AI, Hagmaier R. The Familial Atypical Multiple Mole Melanoma (FAMMM)-Pancreatic Carcinoma (PC) Syndrome. Inherited Cancer Syndromes: Springer New York; 2010. pp. 135-144

[39] Kanth P, Grimmett J, Champine M, Burt R, Samadder NJ. Hereditary colorectal polyposis and cancer syndromes: A primer on diagnosis and management. The American Journal of Gastroenterology. 2017;**112**(10):1509-1525

[40] Syngal S, Brand RE, Church JM, Giardiello FM, Hampel HL, Burt RW. ACG clinical guideline: Genetic testing and management of hereditary gastrointestinal cancer syndromes. 2015;**110**(2):223-262

[41] Malkin D. Li-fraumeni syndrome. Genes & Cancer. 2011;**2**(4):475-484

[42] Conrad C, Fernández-Del CC. Preoperative evaluation and management of the pancreatic head mass. Journal of Surgical Oncology. 2013;**107**(1):23-32

[43] Kanno A, Masamune A, Hanada K, Maguchi H, Shimizu Y, Ueki T, et al. Multicenter study of early pancreatic cancer in Japan. Pancreatology: Official Journal of the International Association of Pancreatology (IAP) [et al.]. 2018;**18**(1):61-67

[44] Pasanen PA, Eskelinen M, Partanen K, Pikkarainen P, Penttilä I, Alhava E. A prospective study of the

value of imaging, serum markers and their combination in the diagnosis of pancreatic carcinoma in symptomatic patients. Anticancer Research. 1992;**12**(6b):2309-2314

[45] Ashida R, Tanaka S, Yamanaka H, Okagaki S, Nakao K, Fukuda J, et al. The Role of Transabdominal Ultrasound in the Diagnosis of Early Stage Pancreatic Cancer: Review and Single-Center Experience. Diagnostics (Basel, Switzerland). 2018;9(1).

[46] Brennan DD, Zamboni GA, Raptopoulos VD, Kruskal JB. Comprehensive preoperative assessment of pancreatic adenocarcinoma with 64-section volumetric CT. Radiographics: A Review Publication of the Radiological Society of North America, Inc. 2007;**27**(6):1653-1666

[47] Fletcher JG, Wiersema MJ, Farrell MA, Fidler JL, Burgart LJ, Koyama T, et al. Pancreatic malignancy: Value of arterial, pancreatic, and hepatic phase imaging with multi-detector row CT. Radiology. 2003;**229**(1):81-90

[48] Sahani DV, Bonaffini PA, Catalano OA, Guimaraes AR, Blake MA. State-of-the-art PET/CT of the pancreas: Current role and emerging indications. Radiographics: A Review Publication of the Radiological Society of North America, Inc. 2012;**32**(4):1133-1158 (discussion 58-60)

[49] Niederau C, Grendell JH. Diagnosis of pancreatic carcinoma. Imaging techniques and tumor markers. Pancreas. 1992;7(1):66-86

[50] Adamek HE, Albert J, Breer H, Weitz M, Schilling D, Riemann JF. Pancreatic cancer detection with magnetic resonance cholangiopancreatography and endoscopic retrograde cholangiopancreatography: A prospective controlled study. Lancet (London, England). 2000;**356**(9225):190-193

[51] Lopez Hänninen E, Amthauer H, Hosten N, Ricke J, Böhmig M, Langrehr J, et al. Prospective evaluation of pancreatic tumors: Accuracy of MR imaging with MR cholangiopancreatography and MR angiography. Radiology. 2002;**224**(1):34-41

[52] Dewitt J, Devereaux BM, Lehman GA, Sherman S, Imperiale TF. Comparison of endoscopic ultrasound and computed tomography for the preoperative evaluation of pancreatic cancer: A systematic review. Clinical Gastroenterology and Hepatology: The Official Clinical Practice Journal of the American Gastroenterological Association. 2006;**4**(6):717-725 quiz 664

[53] Li Y, Jin H, Liao D, Qian B, Zhang Y, Xu M, et al. Contrast-enhanced harmonic endoscopic ultrasonography for the differential diagnosis of pancreatic masses: A systematic review and meta-analysis. Molecular and Clinical Oncology. 2019;**11**(4):425-433

[54] Rahman MIO, Chan BPH, Far PM, Mbuagbaw L, Thabane L, Yaghoobi M. Endoscopic ultrasound versus computed tomography in determining the resectability of pancreatic cancer: A diagnostic test accuracy meta-analysis. Saudi Journal of Gastroenterology: Official Journal of the Saudi Gastroenterology Association. 2020;**26**(3):113-119

[55] Canto MI, Goggins M, Hruban RH, Petersen GM, Giardiello FM, Yeo C, et al. Screening for early pancreatic neoplasia in high-risk individuals: A prospective controlled study. Clinical Gastroenterology and Hepatology: The Official Clinical Practice Journal of the American Gastroenterological Association. 2006;**4**(6):766-781 quiz 665

[56] Canto MI, Harinck F, Hruban RH, Offerhaus GJ, Poley J-W, Kamel I, et al. International Cancer of the Pancreas Screening (CAPS) Consortium summit on the management of patients with increased risk for familial pancreatic cancer. 2013;**62**(3):339-347

[57] Hayashi A, Fan J, Chen R, Ho YJ, Makohon-Moore AP, Lecomte N, et al. A unifying paradigm for transcriptional heterogeneity and squamous features in pancreatic ductal adenocarcinoma. Nature Cancer. 2020;**1**(1):59-74

[58] Pandharipande PV, Heberle C, Dowling EC, Kong CY, Tramontano A, Perzan KE, et al. Targeted screening of individuals at high risk for pancreatic cancer: Results of a simulation model. Radiology. 2015;**275**(1):177-187

[59] NCC N. The NCCN Clinical Practice Guidelines in Oncology (NCCN Guidelines®): Pancreatic Adenocarcinoma. 2019 version 1.2020

[60] Xing H, Wang J, Wang Y, Tong M, Hu H, Huang C, et al. Diagnostic value of CA 19-9 and carcinoembryonic antigen for pancreatic cancer: A meta-analysis. Gastroenterology Research and Practice. 2018;**2018**:8704751

[61] Pasanen PA, Eskelinen M, Partanen K, Pikkarainen P, Penttilä I, Alhava E. Clinical evaluation of a new serum tumour marker CA 242 in pancreatic carcinoma. British Journal of Cancer. 1992;**65**(5):731-734

[62] Gu YL, Lan C, Pei H, Yang SN, Liu YF, Xiao LL. Applicative value of serum CA19-9, CEA, CA125 and CA242 in diagnosis and prognosis for patients with pancreatic cancer treated by concurrent chemoradiotherapy. Asian Pacific Journal of Cancer Prevention. 2015;**16**(15):6569-6573

[63] Abdelrahim M, Esmail A, Xu J, Katz TA, Sharma S, Kalashnikova E, et al. Early relapse detection and monitoring disease status in patients with early-stage pancreatic adenocarcinoma using circulating tumor DNA. The Journal of Surgical Research. 2021;**4**:602-615

[64] Xie ZB, Yao L, Jin C, Fu DL. Circulating tumor cells in pancreatic cancer patients: Efficacy in diagnosis and value in prognosis. Discovery Medicine. 2016;**22**(120):121-128

[65] Herreros-Villanueva M, Bujanda L. Non-invasive biomarkers in pancreatic cancer diagnosis: What we need versus what we have. Annals of Translational Medicine. 2016;**4**(7):134

[66] Kim JE, Lee KT, Lee JK, Paik SW, Rhee JC, Choi KW. Clinical usefulness of carbohydrate antigen 19-9 as a screening test for pancreatic cancer in an asymptomatic population. Journal of Gastroenterology and Hepatology. 2004;**19**(2):182-186

[67] Ballehaninna UK, Chamberlain RS. The clinical utility of serum CA 19-9 in the diagnosis, prognosis and management of pancreatic adenocarcinoma: An evidence based appraisal. Journal of Gastrointestinal Oncology. 2012;**3**(2):105-119

[68] Hao C, Zhang G, Zhang L. Serum CEA levels in 49 different types of cancer and noncancer diseases. Progress in Molecular Biology and Translational Science. 2019;**162**:213-227

[69] Meng Q, Shi S, Liang C, Xiang J, Liang D, Zhang B, et al. Diagnostic accuracy of a CA125-based biomarker panel in patients with pancreatic cancer: A systematic review and meta-analysis. Journal of Cancer. 2017;**8**(17):3615-3622

[70] Haglund C. Tumour marker antigen CA125 in pancreatic cancer: A comparison with CA19-9 and CEA. British Journal of Cancer. 1986;**54**(6):897-901

[71] Yin BW, Lloyd KO. Molecular cloning of the CA125 ovarian cancer antigen: Identification as a new mucin, MUC16. The Journal of Biological Chemistry. 2001;**276**(29):27371-27375

[72] Lei XF, Jia SZ, Ye J, Qiao YL, Zhao GM, Li XH, et al. Application values of detection of serum CA199, CA242 and CA50 in the diagnosis of pancreatic cancer. Journal of Biological Regulators and Homeostatic Agents. 2017;**31**(2):383-388

[73] Dou H, Sun G, Zhang L. Chapter twelve—CA242 as a biomarker for pancreatic cancer and other diseases. In: Zhang L, editor. Progress in Molecular Biology and Translational Science. 162: Academic Press; 2019. pp. 229-239

[74] Dai C, Cao Q, Jiang M, Sun MJ. Serum immunoglobulin G4 in discriminating autoimmune pancreatitis from pancreatic cancer: A diagnostic meta-analysis. Pancreas. 2018;**47**(3):280-284

[75] Ghazale A, Chari ST, Smyrk TC, Levy MJ, Topazian MD, Takahashi N, et al. Value of serum IgG4 in the diagnosis of autoimmune pancreatitis and in distinguishing it from pancreatic cancer. Official Journal of the American College of Gastroenterology. 2007;**102**(8)

[76] Aronsson L, Andersson R, Bauden M, Andersson B, Bygott T, Ansari D. High-density and targeted glycoproteomic profiling of serum proteins in pancreatic cancer and intraductal papillary mucinous neoplasm. Scandinavian Journal of Gastroenterology. 2018;**53**(12):1597-1603

[77] Liu Y, Wang C, Wang R, Wu Y, Zhang L, Liu BF, et al. Isomer-specific profiling of N-glycans derived from human serum for potential biomarker discovery in pancreatic cancer. Journal of Proteomics. 2018;**181**:160-169

[78] Wolrab D, Jirásko R, Cífková E, Höring M, Mei D, Chocholoušková M, et al. Lipidomic profiling of human serum enables detection of pancreatic cancer. Nature Communications. 2022;**13**(1):124

[79] Tien YW, Kuo HC, Ho BI, Chang MC, Chang YT, Cheng MF, et al. A high circulating tumor cell count in portal vein predicts liver metastasis from periampullary or pancreatic cancer: A high portal venous CTC count predicts liver metastases. Medicine. 2016;**95**(16):e3407

[80] Buscail E, Alix-Panabières C, Quincy P, Cauvin T, Chauvet A, Degrandi O, et al. High clinical value of liquid biopsy to detect circulating tumor cells and tumor exosomes in pancreatic ductal adenocarcinoma patients eligible for up-front surgery. Cancers. 2019;**11**(11):7-11

[81] Brancaccio M, Natale F, Falco G, Angrisano T. Cell-free DNA methylation: The new frontiers of pancreatic cancer biomarkers' discovery. 2020;**11**(1):14

[82] Jaworski JJ, Morgan RD, Sivakumar S. Circulating cell-free tumour DNA for early detection of pancreatic cancer. Cancers. 2020;**12**(12):3-9

[83] Sausen M, Phallen J, Adleff V, Jones S, Leary RJ, Barrett MT, et al. Clinical implications of genomic alterations in the tumour and circulation of pancreatic cancer patients. Nature Communications. 2015;**6**:7686

[84] Bettegowda C, Sausen M, Leary RJ, Kinde I, Wang Y, Agrawal N, et al.

Detection of circulating tumor DNA in early- and late-stage human malignancies. Science Translational Medicine. 2014;**6**(224):224ra24

[85] De Guire V, Robitaille R, Tétreault N, Guérin R, Ménard C, Bambace N, et al. Circulating miRNAs as sensitive and specific biomarkers for the diagnosis and monitoring of human diseases: Promises and challenges. Clinical Biochemistry. 2013;**46**(10):846-860

[86] Yu J, Li A, Hong SM, Hruban RH, Goggins M. MicroRNA alterations of pancreatic intraepithelial neoplasias. Clinical Cancer Research: An Official Journal of the American Association for Cancer Research. 2012;**18**(4):981-992

[87] Allenson K, Castillo J, San Lucas FA, Scelo G, Kim DU, Bernard V, et al. High prevalence of mutant KRAS in circulating exosome-derived DNA from early-stage pancreatic cancer patients. Annals of Oncology. 2017;**28**(4):741-747

[88] Melo SA, Luecke LB, Kahlert C, Fernandez AF, Gammon ST, Kaye J, et al. Glypican-1 identifies cancer exosomes and detects early pancreatic cancer. Nature. 2015;**523**(7559):177-182

[89] Versteijne E, van Dam JL, Suker M, Janssen QP, Groothuis K, Akkermans-Vogelaar JM, et al. Neoadjuvant chemoradiotherapy versus upfront surgery for resectable and borderline resectable pancreatic cancer: Long-term results of the Dutch randomized PREOPANC trial. Journal of Clinical Oncology: Official Journal of the American Society of Clinical Oncology. 2022;**40**(11):1220-1230

[90] Ryan DP, Hong TS, Bardeesy N. Pancreatic adenocarcinoma. The New England Journal of Medicine. 2014;**371**(11):1039-1049

[91] Kendrick ML, Cusati D. Total laparoscopic pancreaticoduodenectomy: Feasibility and outcome in an early experience. Archives of Surgery (Chicago, Ill: 1960). 2010;**145**(1):19-23

[92] Palanivelu C, Jani K, Senthilnathan P, Parthasarathi R, Rajapandian S, Madhankumar MV. Laparoscopic pancreaticoduodenectomy: Technique and outcomes. Journal of the American College of Surgeons. 2007;**205**(2):222-230

[93] Kleeff J, Diener MK, Z'Graggen K, Hinz U, Wagner M, Bachmann J, et al. Distal pancreatectomy: Risk factors for surgical failure in 302 consecutive cases. Annals of Surgery. 2007;**245**(4):573-582

[94] Bineshfar N, Malekpour Alamdari N, Rostami T, Mirahmadi A, Zeinalpour A. The effect of preoperative biliary drainage on postoperative complications of pancreaticoduodenectomy: A triple center retrospective study. BMC Surgery. 2022;**22**(1):399

[95] Wang Q, Gurusamy KS, Lin H, Xie X, Wang C. Preoperative biliary drainage for obstructive jaundice. The Cochrane Database of Systematic Reviews. 2008;(3):CD005444

[96] van der Gaag NA, Rauws EA, van Eijck CH, Bruno MJ, van der Harst E, Kubben FJ, et al. Preoperative biliary drainage for cancer of the head of the pancreas. The New England Journal of Medicine. 2010;**362**(2):129-137

[97] Greco SH, August DA, Shah MM, Chen C, Moore DF, Masanam M, et al. Neoadjuvant therapy is associated with lower margin positivity rates after pancreaticoduodenectomy in T1 and T2 pancreatic head cancers: An analysis of the National Cancer Database. Surgery Open Science. 2021;**3**:22-28

[98] Versteijne E, Vogel JA, Besselink MG, Busch ORC, Wilmink JW, Daams JG, et al. Meta-analysis comparing upfront surgery with neoadjuvant treatment in patients with resectable or borderline resectable pancreatic cancer. The British Journal of Surgery. 2018;**105**(8):946-958

[99] Heinrich S, Schäfer M, Weber A, Hany TF, Bhure U, Pestalozzi BC, et al. Neoadjuvant chemotherapy generates a significant tumor response in resectable pancreatic cancer without increasing morbidity: Results of a prospective phase II trial. Annals of Surgery. 2008;**248**(6):1014-1022

[100] Oba A, Ho F, Bao QR, Al-Musawi MH, Schulick RD, Del Chiaro M. Neoadjuvant treatment in pancreatic cancer. Frontiers in Oncology. 2020;**10**:245

[101] Colucci G, Giuliani F, Gebbia V, Biglietto M, Rabitti P, Uomo G, et al. Gemcitabine alone or with cisplatin for the treatment of patients with locally advanced and/or metastatic pancreatic carcinoma: A prospective, randomized phase III study of the Gruppo Oncologia dell'Italia Meridionale. Cancer. 2002;**94**(4):902-910

[102] Scheithauer W, Schüll B, Ulrich-Pur H, Schmid K, Raderer M, Haider K, et al. Biweekly high-dose gemcitabine alone or in combination with capecitabine in patients with metastatic pancreatic adenocarcinoma: A randomized phase II trial. Annals of Oncology: Official Journal of the European Society for Medical Oncology. 2003;**14**(1):97-104

[103] Tempero M, Plunkett W, Ruiz Van Haperen V, Hainsworth J, Hochster H, Lenzi R, et al. Randomized phase II comparison of dose-intense gemcitabine: Thirty-minute infusion and fixed dose rate infusion in patients with pancreatic adenocarcinoma. Journal of Clinical Oncology: Official Journal of the American society of Clinical Oncology. 2003;**21**(18):3402-3408

[104] Von Hoff DD, Ervin T, Arena FP, Chiorean EG, Infante J, Moore M, et al. Increased survival in pancreatic cancer with nab-paclitaxel plus gemcitabine. The New England Journal of Medicine. 2013;**369**(18):1691-1703

[105] Conroy T, Desseigne F, Ychou M, Bouché O, Guimbaud R, Bécouarn Y, et al. FOLFIRINOX versus gemcitabine for metastatic pancreatic cancer. The New England Journal of Medicine. 2011;**364**(19):1817-1825

Chapter 6

Surgical Options to Mitigate the Consequences of Pancreatic Anastomosis Leak after Pancreaticoduodenectomy

Azize Saroglu and Alexander Julianov

Abstract

Pancreaticoduodenectomy is still the only treatment option that offers a chance to cure patients with pancreatic cancer and malignant periampullary tumors. Pancreaticojejunal anastomosis is the preferred method of reconstruction after pancreaticoduodenectomy. However, because of the high incidence of anastomotic leak and subsequent severe consequences, pancreaticojejunal anastomosis still remains the Achilles' heel of the operation. Several technical modifications of pancreaticojejunal anastomosis exist, but none completely eliminates anastomotic leak, postoperative pancreatic fistula, or severe complications. Therefore, considerable efforts have been made to study and develop surgical options that can mitigate the severity and avoid fatal consequences of postoperative pancreatic fistula. This chapter presents and discusses some of the existing and emerging surgical strategies devoted to mitigating the catastrophic consequences of pancreatic anastomotic leaks.

Keywords: pancreaticoduodenectomy, anastomotic leak, pancreatic fistula, pancreaticojejunostomy, pancreatic cancer, falciform ligament, transanastomotic external stent, coronary stent

1. Introduction

Pancreaticoduodenectomy (PD) is still the only treatment option that offers a chance to cure patients with pancreatic cancer and malignant periampullary tumors. Regarding the constantly growing incidence of pancreatic ductal adenocarcinoma [1, 2], the demand for PD worldwide is expected to increase as well. Pioneer surgeons such as Codivilla in 1898 and Kausch in 1909 performed the first pancreatic head resections without pancreatic anastomosis [3, 4]. Whipple also performed his first PD without reconstruction of pancreatico-enteric continuity [5], but in his subsequent 36 pancreatic head resections reconstructed the drainage of the pancreatic duct by pancreaticojejunal anastomosis (PJA), which is now the preferred method to reestablish pancreatic ductal drainage.

Currently, PD remains a complex and risky surgical intervention, requiring substantial surgeon experience despite advances in surgical techniques and technology [6, 7]. With the refinement of the surgical technique of PD, the main problems with intraoperative bleeding and early postoperative mortality were gradually resolved, and a series of more than a hundred consecutive operations with no postoperative mortality were published for the first time in the 90s from the leading centers [8, 9]. However, compared to other abdominal operations, the complication rate of PD is still high, mainly due to PJA leak and subsequent severe consequences that remain the Achilles' heel of the operation. It becomes obvious that searching for a no-leak PJA technique is unrealistic, and it is considered that an individual surgeon's mastery of a specific anastomotic technique, in conjunction with a large personal experience, is likely to be the best predictor of a low PJA leak rate [10–12].

2. Surgical techniques to mitigate the consequences of PJA leak

The main problem of a leaked PJA comes from the extravasation of pancreatic enzyme-rich juice into the perianastomotic region, which can cause severe morbidity due to the development of intra-abdominal abscesses leading to sepsis or pseudoaneurysms leading to severe hemorrhage and even mortality. Surgical techniques devoted to mitigating the fatal consequences of PJA leak aim to control/reduce pancreatic juice extravasation into the abdomen or to prevent the contact of dissected peripancreatic vascular structures with leaked pancreatic enzymes, decreasing the incidence and grade of postoperative pancreatic fistula (POPF) (**Figure 1**).

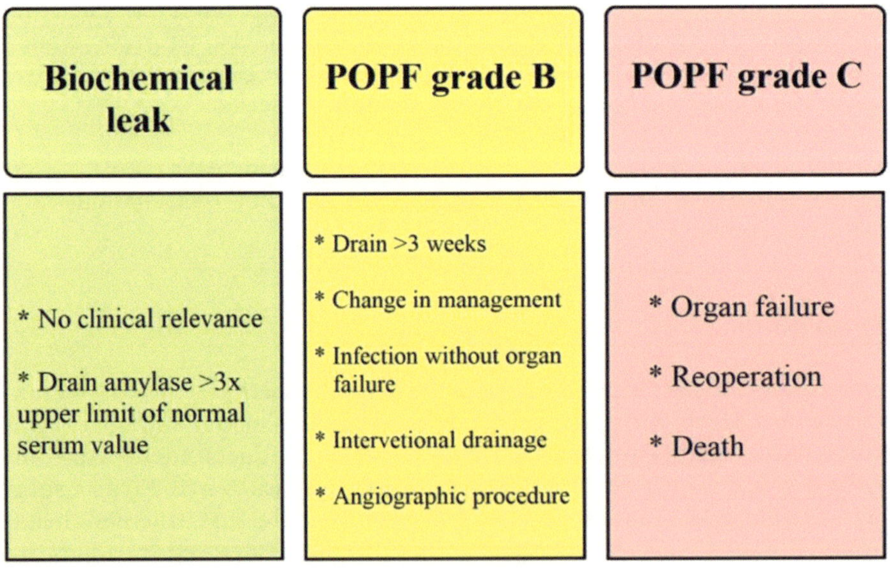

Figure 1.
International Study Group of Pancreatic Surgery (ISGPS) grading of postoperative pancreatic fistula (modified by [13]).

2.1 Transanastomotic external pancreatic duct stent

The goal of transanastomotic external stenting is to control pancreatic juice leakage by diverting the pancreatic secretion through the PJA outside the body by exteriorization of the stent from the jejunal lumen through a Witzel tunnel (**Figure 2**).

From a technical standpoint, we performed duct-to-mucosa PJA in two layers and opened the jejunum corresponding to the pancreatic duct after completion of the external layer of the posterior row sutures of the anastomosis. The posterior duct-to-mucosa sutures are then easily placed, and the chosen transanastomotic stent is introduced through a small opening in the jejunal limb at a distance of approximately 10 cm from the PJA. We left the uncut and used at least one of the tied posterior row duct-to-mucosa sutures to secure the stent in the desired position. The PJA is completed then, and the stent is secured at a second point in the Witzel tunnel. It is also important to note that some measures have to be taken in order to divert or reduce the flow of the pancreatic juice in the operative field after transection of the gland, as it might cause intraperitoneal saponification around the pancreas due to pancreatic lipase-induced lipolysis, and has been shown to negatively impact anastomotic healing [14]. As a preventive measure, we temporarily placed the external stent in the remnant pancreatic duct (**Figure 3**) and/or covered the cut surface of the pancreas with gauze.

The use of transanastomotic external stents after PD has been a matter of debate and controversy due to conflicting results published from single-institution retrospective and/or nonrandomized studies. However, initial randomized trials on the subject clearly demonstrated the ability of the technique to reduce morbidity and the incidence of clinically relevant PJA leaks, especially in patients at high risk of developing POPF [15–17]. Further research and high-quality evidence from systematic reviews and meta-analyses have confirmed the efficacy of transanastomotic external stents in reducing the incidence and grade of POPF in both randomized and nonrandomized settings [18–21]. The largest systematic review to date with meta-analysis of the POPF-related mortality rate includes 60,739 patients and undoubtedly confirmed that external transanastomotic stents decreased the POPF-related mortality rate [22].

The main problems with the use of external stents are stent malfunction and/or migration. Stent migration can be prevented by securing the stent at least at two

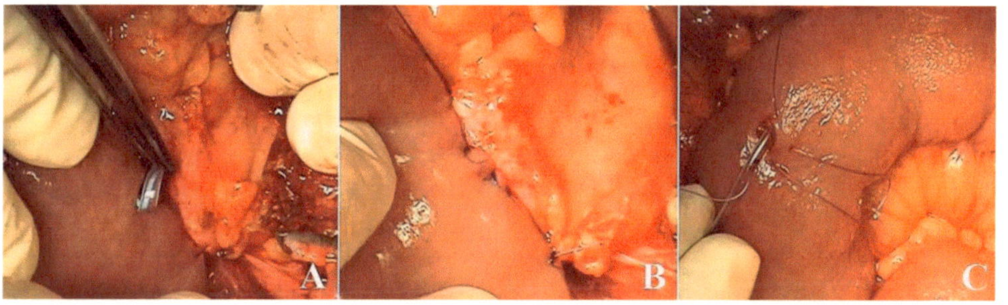

Figure 2.
Pancreaticoduodenectomy. Transanastomotic stent placement. (A) Positioning the stent after completion of the posterior row sutures of the PJA. (B) Stent covered by anterior, first row, and duct-to-mucosa sutures. (C) Exteriorization of the stent from the jejunal lumen [original photograph].

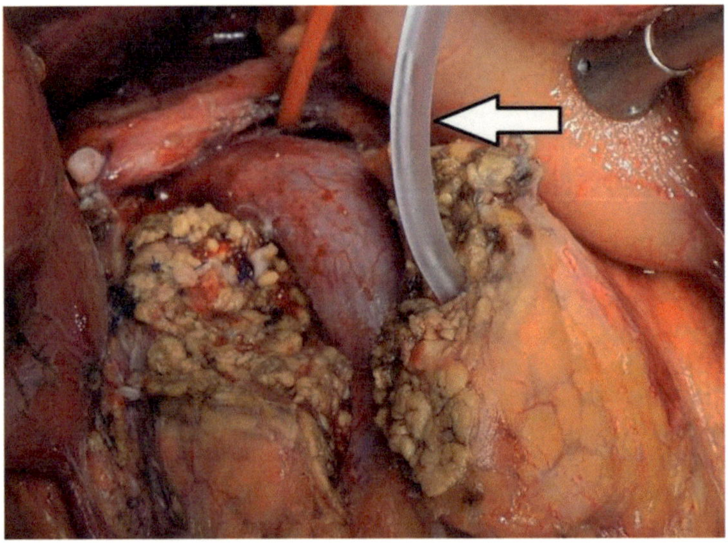

Figure 3.
Pancreaticoduodenectomy. Stent (arrow) is placed in the pancreatic duct immediately after transection of the gland to divert the pancreatic juice from the operative field during the resection [original photograph].

points: at the anastomosis and at the Witzel tunnel, and by leaving the ample length of the stent between the Witzel tunnel and abdominal wall to compensate for the tension of the fixation point at the anastomosis in a case of abdominal distension during the postoperative period. Malfunction of nondisplaced stents is rare and is a result of clotting (which can be resolved by stent irrigation) or of use of a stent with just 1–2 distal openings that could impact the pancreatic duct if positioned too distally from the PJA. To prevent the latter, additional holes can be made in the stent tube to secure drainage of the duct close to the PJA. However, we consider that even the displaced from the pancreatic duct external stent can still be beneficial by reducing the intraluminal pressure of the jejunal limb in cases of PJA leak.

2.2 Transanastomotic internal pancreatic duct stent

The internal transanastomotic stent seems theoretically superior to the external stent, as it eliminates the exteriorized part of the drain. However, the results of numerous randomized trials, systematic reviews, and meta-analyses failed to prove the benefit of internal PJA stents versus no-stent in terms of the incidence and severity of POPF, morbidity, and mortality after PD [18, 19, 21–25]. The use of internal stents is associated with a high rate of stent migration, and, contrary to an external stent, the malfunction of an internal stent in place cannot be assessed.

As the theoretical benefits of internal PJA stents cannot be neglected, recent research has focused on the options to find/develop an internal stent that can be safely positioned and secured in place, especially in a patient with a soft pancreas and very small duct size, in whom the use of an external stent is impractical because of the very narrow lumen of the fitting stent or even impossible. To overcome these limitations in patients with a small pancreatic duct size that cannot fit the external stent, since November 2016 we started to use as an internal PJA stent a commercially available, covered, and balloon-expandable coronary artery stent (**Figure 4**).

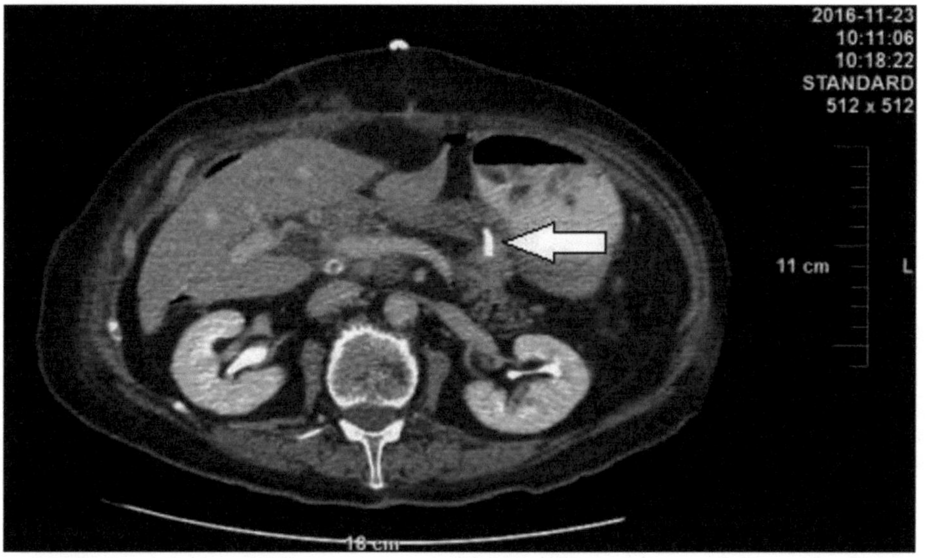

Figure 4.
Pancreaticoduodenectomy. Postoperative computed tomography showing pancreaticojejunal anastomosis with covered coronary artery stent (arrow) in place [original photograph].

We positioned the stent using the over-the-wire technique after completion of the posterior row sutures of the PJA. Briefly, the jejunal limb was punctured at a chosen point opposite the transected pancreatic duct with the needle passing through both the lateral and medial bowel walls. A guidewire was inserted through the needle into the pancreatic duct. The coronary artery stent is positioned under intraoperative ultrasound guidance over the wire in the anastomosis and the pancreatic duct and expanded enough to be self-impacted in the duct. Anastomosis was then completed using anterior row sutures. A similar use of an uncovered coronary artery stent with positioning under X-ray guidance was recently reported by Huscher et al. [26], and the use of biodegradable stents in 10 patients was reported by Sulieman et al. [27]. Although the use of expandable internal PJA stents is still in its infancy, the initial results of their use are promising in terms of reducing the clinically relevant POPF rate and major morbidity with no stent-related complications [26, 27].

2.3 Peripancreatic vessel wrap

Irrespective of the anastomotic technique and use of transanastomotic stents, the risk of high-grade POPF is not negligible, especially for International Study Group of Pancreatic Surgery (ISGPS) grade C-D anastomoses (**Figure 5**).

The most dramatic and life-threatening complication of PJA leak is grade C POPF with severe postoperative hemorrhage caused by erosion of a major peripancreatic vessel from the leaked pancreatic juice and accompanying local infection. Different surgical options can be used to wrap the peripancreatic vessels in an attempt to prevent contact with aggressive leakage content in the case of POPF, thus preventing vessel erosion and severe hemorrhage. For this purpose, we routinely use the teres/falciform ligament of the liver (**Figure 6**), which is carefully preserved and tailored during laparotomy at the beginning of the surgery. Alternatively, omental or peritoneal patches can be used to protect the vessels in the case of a sacrificed or small teres

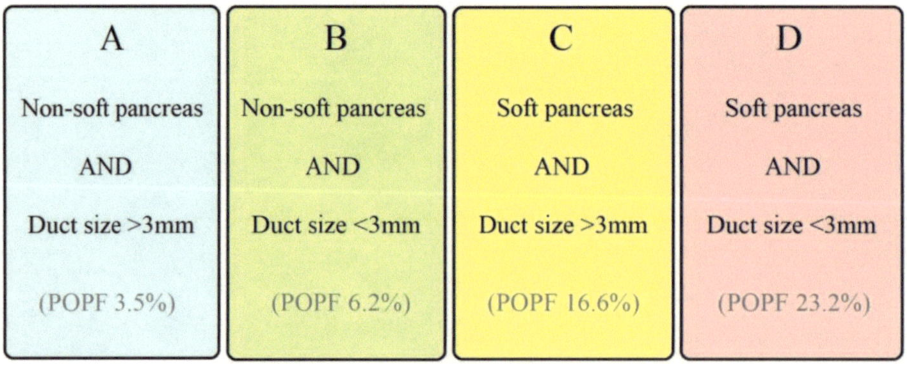

Figure 5.
Clinically relevant postoperative pancreatic fistula (POPF) rates for ISGPS A-D grades of pancreaticojejunal anastomoses (modified by [28]).

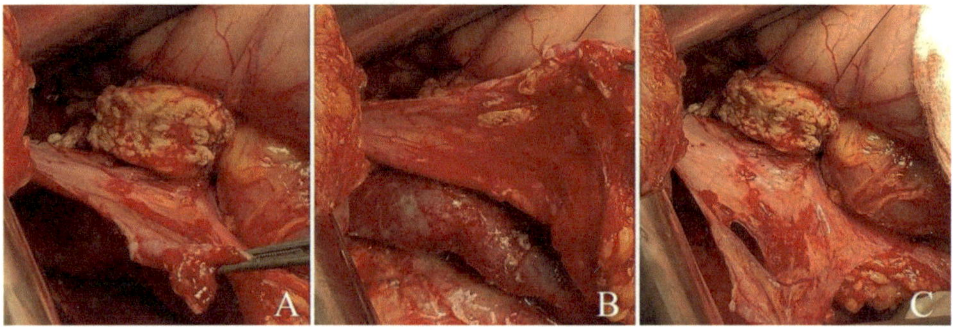

Figure 6.
Pancreaticoduodenectomy. (A–C) Wrapping the retroperitoneal vessels with the teres/falciform ligament flap [original photograph].

ligament. The chosen wrap is carefully positioned to cover the major arteries and veins and secured in place with nonabsorbable sutures. From the above options for the protection of divided or skeletonized vessels, the use of a teres/falciform ligament has become the most frequently applied technique due to evidence for its effectiveness in published case series [29–33], systematic reviews [34–36], and a recent randomized clinical trial [37].

2.4 Prophylactic abdominal drainage

Historically, abdominal drains are routinely placed at the time of pancreatic resection to allow postoperative evacuation of intra-abdominal secretions, lymphatic fluid, blood, bile, and pancreatic juice. Theoretically, the use of drains should reduce the incidence of intra-abdominal collections and the need for re-intervention after PD. However, the routine use of prophylactic abdominal drains after PD has been questioned in the past decade and remains a matter of debate and controversy [38–41]. Further randomized clinical trials on the subject also reported conflicting results and did not resolve this issue. The PANDRA trial concluded that clinically important POPF was significantly reduced in patients without drainage, although there was no significant difference in overall morbidity [38]. However, the next randomized trial was prematurely closed because patients without prophylactic intraperitoneal drainage had a higher mortality rate than those with drainage [39]. Subsequent systematic reviews and meta-analyses also reported that patients without prophylactic drainage after PD had a higher mortality rate despite a similar or lower rate of overall major complications and readmissions [40, 41]. Regarding the above data, although the use of prophylactic abdominal drains in PD is associated with a higher rate of POPF compared to no drain abandoning, its routine use is not justified. Moreover, there is still room for research, and not well-studied options, to achieve more benefits from prophylactic drains to reduce the incidence and grade of clinically relevant POPF after PD. For this purpose, a few groups have reported promising results with prophylactic saline irrigation around a PJA after PD and around the pancreatic stump after distal pancreatectomy [42–44].

We routinely place prophylactic drains parallel to the upper and lower borders of the remnant pancreas, passing the drains to the right, beneath the PJA, and hepaticojejunostomy. In the case of a biochemical leak, we started intermittent drain irrigation (2–3 times daily with 20–30 ml saline solution per drain with no suction) to dilute the aggressive content of the subclinical leak. In our experience, this strategy was always effective in controlling the leak and maintaining the drain patent.

3. Conclusion

The constant evolution of pancreatic surgery makes PD a widespread intervention, which is now performed routinely even outside specialized centers. Although there are several reports of reduced intra-abdominal complications and mortality, POPF remains the most common unavoidable and life-threatening complication of PD. It becomes obvious that no single measure could be effective enough to eliminate POPF or to reduce its severity to the level of clinically irrelevant postoperative events. However, the combined use of the existing and emerging surgical strategies proved to mitigate the catastrophic consequences of pancreatic anastomosis leak and might be more successful in attempts to achieve this goal.

Based on available clinical evidence, we routinely used a combination of the above-mentioned surgical measures (transanastomotic drain plus vessel wrap plus abdominal drains) in more than a hundred pancreatic resections. Our postoperative protocol included daily measurement of drain fluid amylase levels and prompt start of drain irrigation in a case of biochemical leak, as mentioned above. We proceeded with irrigation of the drain until normalization of the drain fluid amylase (less than 3× the upper limit of normal serum amylase), but no longer after the second postoperative week. A systemic antibiotic is started if the patient develops a clinically apparent PJA leak, body temperature >37.5°C, or had prior chemotherapy. The biochemical leak rate was 17% and the ISGPS grade B POPF rate was 11%, with no POPF-related mortality. Notably, none of the patients in this series developed ISGPS grade C POPF nor required image-guided intervention or reoperation. Although none of the surgical techniques can completely eliminate the occurrence of PJA leak after PD, the simultaneous use of measures proven to reduce the risk and/or severity of POPF can effectively mitigate the catastrophic consequences of pancreatic anastomosis leak and should be implemented in PD management protocols.

Conflict of interest

The authors declare no conflict of interest.

Abbreviations

PD	pancreaticoduodenectomy
PJA	pancreaticojejunal anastomosis
POPF	postoperative pancreatic fistula
ISGPS	International Study Group of Pancreatic Surgery

Author details

Azize Saroglu* and Alexander Julianov
Trakia Hospital, Stara Zagora, Bulgaria

*Address all correspondence to: azize_saroglu@hotmail.com

References

[1] Ilic M, Ilic I. Epidemiology of pancreatic cancer. World Journal of Gastroenterology. 2016;**22**:9694-9705. DOI: 10.3748/wjg.v22.i44.9694

[2] Rawla P, Sunkara T, Gaduputic V. Epidemiology of pancreatic cancer: Global trends, etiology and risk factors. World Journal of Oncology. 2019;**10**: 10-27. DOI: 10.14740/wjon1166

[3] Schnelldorfer T, Sarr MG. Alessandro Codivilla and the first pancreatoduodenectomy. Archives of Surgery. 2009;**144**:1179-1184. DOI: 10.1001/archsurg.2009.219

[4] Griffin JF, Poruk KE, Wolfgang CL. Pancreatic cancer surgery: Past, present, and future. Chinese Journal of Cancer Research. 2015;**27**:332-348. DOI: 10.3978/j.issn.1000-9604.2015.06.07

[5] Are C, Dhir M, Ravipati L. History of pancreaticoduodenectomy: Early misconceptions, initial milestones and the pioneers. HPB. 2011;**13**:377-384. DOI: 10.1111/j.1477-2574.2011.00305.x

[6] Aziz H, Khan M, Khan S, Serra GP, Goodman MD, Genyk Y, et al. Assessing the perioperative complications and outcomes of robotic pancreaticoduodenectomy using the national cancer database: Is it ready for prime time? Journal of Robotic Surgery. 2022;**16**:687-694. DOI: 10.1007/s11701-021-01296-3

[7] McMillan MT, Zureikat AH, Hogg ME, Kowalsky SJ, Zeh HJ, Sprys MH, et al. A propensity score-matched analysis of robotic vs open pancreatoduodenectomy on incidence of pancreatic fistula. JAMA Surgery. 2017;**152**:327-335. DOI: 10.1001/jamasurg.2016.4755

[8] Trede M, Schwall G, Saeger HD. Survival after pancreatoduodenectomy. 118 Consecutive resections without an operative mortality. Annals of Surgery. 1990;**211**:447-458. DOI: 10.1097/00000658-199004000-00011

[9] Cameron JL, Pitt HA, Yeo CJ, Lillemoe KD, Kaufman HS, J Coleman J. One hundred and forty-five consecutive pancreaticoduodenectomies without mortality. Annals of Surgery. 1993;**217**:430-435. DOI: 10.1097/00000658-199305010-00002

[10] Ball CG, Howard TJ. Does the type of pancreaticojejunostomy after Whipple alter the leak rate? Advances in Surgery. 2010;**44**:131-148. DOI: 10.1016/j.yasu.2010.05.020

[11] Shrikhande SV, Qureshi SS, Rajneesh N, Shukla PJ. Pancreatic anastomoses after pancreaticoduodenectomy: Do we need further studies? World Journal of Surgery. 2005;**29**:1642-1649. DOI: 10.1007/s00268-005-0137-3

[12] Adams DB. The pancreatic anastomosis: The danger of a leak, which anastomotic technique is better? Journal of Gastrointestinal Surgery. 2009;**13**:1182-1183. DOI: 10.1007/s11605-009-0865-z

[13] Bassi C, Marchegiani G, Dervenis C, Sarr M, Abu Hilal M, Adham M, et al. The 2016 update of the International Study Group (ISGPS) definition and grading of postoperative pancreatic fistula: 11 years after. Surgery. 2017;**161**:584-591. DOI: 10.1016/j.surg.2016.11.014

[14] Sugiura T, Uesaka K, Ashida R, Ohgi K, Okamura Y, Yamada M, et al. Hepatopancreatoduodenectomy with delayed division of the pancreatic parenchyma: A novel technique for reducing pancreatic fistula. Annals of Surgery Open. 2021;**2**:e112. DOI: 10.1097/AS9.0000000000000112

[15] Poon RTP, Fan ST, Lo CM, Ng KK, Yuen WK, Yeung C, et al. External drainage of pancreatic duct with a stent to reduce leakage rate of pancreaticojejunostomy after pancreaticoduodenectomy: A prospective randomized trial. Annals of Surgery. 2007;**246**:425-433. DOI: 10.1097/SLA.0b013e3181492c28

[16] Pessaux P, Sauvanet A, Mariette C, Paye F, Muscari F, Cunha AS, et al. External pancreatic duct stent decreases pancreatic fistula rate after pancreaticoduodenectomy: Prospective multicenter randomized trial. Annals of Surgery. 2011;**253**:879-885. DOI: 10.1097/SLA.0b013e31821219af

[17] Motoi F, Egawa S, Rikiyama T, Katayose Y, Unno M. Randomized clinical trial of external stent drainage of the pancreatic duct to reduce postoperative pancreatic fistula after pancreaticojejunostomy. British Journal of Surgery. 2012;**99**:524-531. DOI: 10.1002/bjs.8654

[18] Wang Q, He XR, Tian JH, Yang KH. Pancreatic duct stents at pancreaticoduodenectomy: A meta-analysis. Digestive Surgery. 2013;**30**:415-424. DOI: 10.1159/000355982

[19] Patel K, Teta A, Sukharamwala P, Thoens J, Szuchmacher M, Peter DVP. External pancreatic duct stent reduces pancreatic fistula: A meta-analysis and systematic review. International Journal of Surgery. 2014;**12**:827-832. DOI: 10.1016/j.ijsu.2014.06.008

[20] Jiang Y, Chen Q, Shao Y, Gao Z, Jin M, Gao B, et al. The prognostic value of external vs internal pancreatic duct stents after pancreaticoduodenectomy in patients with FRS ≥ 4: A retrospective cohort study. BMC Surgery. 2021;**21**:81. DOI: 10.1186/s12893-021-01074-w

[21] Gou C, Xie B, Guo D. Does pancreatic duct stent placement lead to decreased postoperative pancreatic fistula rates after pancreaticoduodenectomy? A meta-analysis. International Journal of Surgery. 2022;**103**:106707. DOI: 10.1016/j.ijsu.2022.106707

[22] Pedrazzoli S. Pancreatoduodenectomy (PD) and postoperative pancreatic fistula (POPF): A systematic review and analysis of the POPF-related mortality rate in 60,739 patients retrieved from the English literature published between 1990 and 2015. Medicine (Baltimore). 2017;**96**:e6858. DOI: 10.1097/MD.0000000000006858

[23] Xiong JJ, Altaf K, Mukherjee R, Huang W, Hu WM, Li A, et al. Systematic review and meta-analysis of outcomes after intraoperative pancreatic duct stent placement during pancreaticoduodenectomy. The British Journal of Surgery. 2012;**99**:1050-1061. DOI: 10.1002/bjs.8788

[24] Dong Z, Xu J, Wang Z, Petrov MS. Stents for the prevention of pancreatic fistula following pancreaticoduodenectomy. Cochrane Database of Systematic Reviews. 2016;**5**:CD008914. DOI: 10.1002/14651858.CD008914.pub3

[25] Jiang Y, Chen Q, Wang Z, Shao Y, Hu C, Ding Y, et al. The prognostic value of external vs internal pancreatic duct stents in CR-POPF after pancreaticoduodenectomy: A systematic review and meta-analysis. Journal of Investigative Surgery. 2021;**34**:738-746. DOI: 10.1080/08941939.2019.1691687

[26] Huscher C, Perri G, Lazzarin G, Marchegiani G, Malleo G, Salvia R, et al. Coronary artery stent for securing high-risk pancreatico-jejunal anastomosis after pancreatoduodenectomy: A pilot series. Annals of Surgery. 2022;**275**:e665-e668. DOI: 10.1097/SLA.0000000000005316

[27] Sulieman I, Elaffandi A, Elmoghazy W, Khalaf H. Use of biodegradable stents in pancreaticoduodenectomy: Initial experience. Surgical Innovation. 23 Sep 2022:15533506221123355. DOI: 10.1177/15533506221123355 [Epub ahead of print]

[28] Schuh F, Mihaljevic AL, Probst P, Trudeau M, Muller PC, Marchegiani G, et al. A simple classification of pancreatic duct size and texture predicts postoperative pancreatic fistula: A classification of the international study group of pancreatic surgery (ISGPS). Annals of Surgery. 12 Mar 2021. DOI: 10.1097/SLA.0000000000004855 [Epub ahead of print]

[29] Abe N, Sugiyama M, Suzuki Y, Yanagida O, Masaki T, Mori T, et al. Falciform ligament in pancreatoduodenectomy for protection of skeletonized and divided vessels. Journal of Hepato-Biliary-Pancreatic Surgery. 2009;**16**:184-188. DOI: 10.1007/s00534-008-0036-8

[30] Ray S, Sanyal S, Ghatak S, Sonar PK, Das S, Khamrui S, et al. Falciform ligament flap for the protection of the gastroduodenal artery stump after pancreaticoduodenectomy: A single center experience. Journal of Visceral Surgery. 2016;**153**(1):9-13. DOI: 10.1016/j.jviscsurg.2015.10.007

[31] Müssle B, Wierick A, Distler M, Weitz J, Welsch T. Falciform ligament wrap for prevention of gastroduodenal artery bleed after pancreatoduodenectomy. The Journal of Surgical Research. 2017;**207**:215-222. DOI: 10.1016/j.jss.2016.08.087

[32] Meng L, Cai H, Cai Y, Li Y, Peng B. Wrapping the stump of the gastroduodenal artery using the ligamentum teres hepatis during laparoscopic pancreaticoduodenectomy: A center's preliminary experience. BMC Surgery. 2021;**21**(1):70. DOI: 10.1186/s12893-021-01076-8

[33] Sakamoto Y, Shimada K, Esaki M, Kajiwara T, Sano T, Kosuge T. Wrapping the stump of the gastroduodenal artery using the falciform ligament during pancreaticoduodenectomy. Journal of the American College of Surgeons. 2007;**204**(2):334-336. DOI: 10.1016/j.jamcollsurg.2006.11.015

[34] Ramia JM, de la Plaza R, Adel F, Ramiro C, Arteaga V, Garcia-Parreño J. Wrapping in pancreatic surgery: A systematic review. ANZ Journal of Surgery. 2014;**84**(12):921-924. DOI: 10.1111/ans.12491

[35] Baskaran V, Banerjee JK, Ghosh SR, Kumar SS, Anand S, Menon G, et al. Applications of hepatic round ligament/falciform ligament flap and graft in abdominal surgery—A review of their utility and efficacy. Langenbeck's Archives of Surgery. 2021;**406**(5):1249-1281. DOI: 10.1007/s00423-020-02031-6

[36] Nour HM, Peristeri DV, Ahsan A, Shafique S, Khan PM, Sajid MS. Regional vessels wrapping following pancreaticoduodenectomy reduces the risk of post-operative extra-luminal bleeding. A systematic review. Annals of Medical Surgery. 2022;**82**:104618. DOI: 10.1016/j.amsu.2022.104618

[37] Welsch T, Müssle B, Korn S, Sturm D, Bork U, Distler M, et al. Pancreatoduodenectomy with or without

prophylactic falciform ligament wrap around the hepatic artery for prevention of postpancreatectomy haemorrhage: Randomized clinical trial (PANDA trial). British Journal of Surgery. 2021;**109**: 37-45. DOI: 10.1093/bjs/znab363

[38] Witzigmann H, Diener MK, Kienkötter S, Rossion I, Bruckner T, Werner B, et al. No need for routine drainage after pancreatic head resection: The Dual-Center, Randomized, Controlled PANDRA Trial (ISRCTN04937707). Annals of Surgery. 2016;**264**:528-537. DOI: 10.1097/SLA.0000000000001859

[39] Van Buren G, Bloomston M, Hughes SJ, Winter J, Behrman SW, Zyromski NJ, et al. A randomized prospective multicenter trial of pancreaticoduodenectomy with and without routine intraperitoneal drainage. Annals of Surgery. 2014;**259**:605-612. DOI: 10.1097/SLA.0000000000000460

[40] Wang YC, Szatmary P, Zhu JQ, Xiong JJ, Huang W, Gomatos I, et al. Prophylactic intra-peritoneal drain placement following pancreaticoduodenectomy: A systematic review and meta-analysis. World Journal of Gastroenterology. 2015;**21**:2510-2521. DOI: 10.3748/wjg.v21.i8.2510

[41] He S, Xia J, Zhang W, Lai M, Cheng N, Liu Z, et al. Prophylactic abdominal drainage for pancreatic surgery. Cochrane Database of Systematic Reviews. 2021;**12**:CD010583. DOI: 10.1002/14651858.CD010583.pub5

[42] Nakano H, Asakura T, Sakurai J, Koizumi S, Asano T, Watanabe T, et al. Prophylactic irrigation around a pancreaticojejunostomy for the treatment of a pancreatic fistula after a pancreaticoduodenectomy in patients with a risky pancreatic remnant. Hepato-Gastroenterology. 2008;**55**:717-721

[43] Bu X, Xu Y, Xu J, Dai X. Continuous irrigation around pancreatic remnant decreases pancreatic fistula-related intraabdominal complications after distal pancreatectomy. Langenbeck's Archives of Surgery. 2013;**398**:1083-1089. DOI: 10.1007/s00423-013-1122-1

[44] Chao J, Zhu C, Jia Z, Zhang X, Qin X. Prophylactic active irrigation drainage reduces the risk of post-operative pancreatic fistula-related complications in patients undergoing limited pancreatic resection. Journal of Minimum Access Surgery. 2021;**17**:197-201. DOI: 10.4103/jmas.JMAS_290_19

Section 4

Pancreatitis in Children

Chapter 7

Acute Pancreatitis in Children with Acute Lymphoblastic Leukemia Using L-Asparaginase: A Review of the Literature

Kmira Zahra, Wided Cherif, Naila Fathallah, Haifa Regaieg, Monia Zaier, Yosra Ben Youssef and Abderrahim Khelif

Abstract

L-asparaginase (L-Aspa) is utilized as a part of the therapy in children with acute lymphoblastic leukemia (ALL), achieving remission in 83–95% of the younger patients. Hypersensitivity reactions, as well as liver and pancreatic cytotoxicity, are severe documented side effects. L-Aspa-induced acute pancreatitis (AP) has been observed in 2.5–16% of treated patients. Patients with mild pancreatitis may be retreated with L-Aspa if they have no clinical symptoms within 48 hours, amylase and lipase levels are less than three times the normal's upper limit, and there is no evidence of pseudocysts or necrosis on imaging. It is crucial to monitor patients under L-Aspa therapy, through careful observation of clinical signs and laboratory follow-up, as well as a continuous checkup for associated medications.

Keywords: acute lymphoblastic leukemia, L-Asparaginase, acute pancreatitis, diagnosis of pancreatits, treatment of pancreatits

1. Introduction

L-Asparaginase (L-Aspa) is a keystone therapy of acute lymphoblastic leukemia (ALL) [1]. Its mechanism of action is complex, depleting the body of the non-essential amino acid asparagine through deamidation of asparagine into aspartic acid and ammonia [2]. The proportion of cured patients under L-Aspa increases by targeting malignant lymphoblasts, which lost the ability to asparagine synthesis [3, 4]. In fact, asparaginase therapy leads to the complete depletion of serum asparagine concentrations, depriving leukemic blasts of this amino acid, resulting in reduced protein synthesis and ultimately leukemic cell death [5]. L-Aspa is administered in combination with other anti-neoplastic drugs intramuscularly or intravenously. However, with a high incidence of cumulative dose of asparaginase ranging from 2 to 10%, L-Aspa-associated pancreatitis is the main cause of substantial morbidity in patients receiving this drug [6]. Despite low mortality, asparaginase-associated pancreatitis (AAP) often results in a switch of asparaginase therapy, which might be associated with an increased risk of leukemia relapse [3, 4].

This review explores the definition, treatment, complications, and possible risk factors for AAP in children.

2. L-Asparaginase (L-Aspa)

2.1 Mechanism of action

Asparagine is a non-essential amino acid, provided from food or produced by asparagine synthetase (ASNS). Normal cells may manufacture L-asparagine for growth using the transaminase enzyme, which converts oxaloacetate into the intermediate aspartate, which then transfers an amino group from glutamate to oxaloacetate, producing ketoglutarate and aspartate. Finally, the enzyme asparagine synthetase transforms aspartate to asparagine in healthy cells [7].

ASNS is very low expressed or even absent in ALL cells, rendering them reliant on extracellular asparagine for growth and survival, L-Aspa lowers plasma asparagine concentrations by catalyzing asparagine deamination into aspartic acid and ammonia [2]. Asparaginase therapy results in the entire depletion of blood asparagine concentrations, depriving leukemic blasts of this amino acid, resulting in decreased protein synthesis and, eventually, leukemic cell death at optimal enzyme activity levels [5].

Circulating asparagine concentrations range between 40 and 80 μm in normal physiological conditions [8]. Researchers defined complete asparagine depletion as less than 0.1–0.2 μm based on the limit of detection of the high-performance liquid chromatography assay used [8, 9]. However, the critical level of serum asparagine depletion for in vivo leukemic cell death is unknown.

2.2 Asparaginase formulations

Three distinct formulations of L-Aspa are available. The native-Asparaginase modified pegylated version (PEG-Asparaginase), are both generated from *Escherichia coli* (*E. coli*). The third is Erwinase, which is derived from *Erwinia Chrysanthemi*. The three formulations vary in terms of pharmacokinetics, pharmacodynamics, and immunogenic propreties [10, 11]. The glutamine pharmacokinetics differs in these current formulations. While both *Erwinia Chrysanthemi* and *E. coli*–derived asparaginase formulations show similar binding affinities for glutamine, the maximal conversion rate at saturation is greater with *Erwinia Chrysanthemi* [12, 13].

First-line treatment in ALL was based on native *E. coli* asparaginase. However, in the United States, this formulation was replaced with PEG-asparaginase [5].

Erwinia asparaginase, which is produced from a distinct bacterial origin, has a unique immunogenic profile, with no cross-reactivity with native *E. coli* asparaginase or PEG-asparaginase [14]. Consequently, *Erwinia* asparaginase is indicated as a component of a multiagent chemotherapy regimen in patients with ALL and a history of hypersensitivity to *E. coli*-derived asparaginases [5].

Intravenously or intramuscularly routes are possible for the three asparaginase formulations. However, the intramuscular route is associated with lower plasma peak values, local bleeding in cases of thrombocytopenia, and local pain, which can be alleviated by co-administration of lidocaine [15]. However, intramuscular injections have the advantage to reduce the risk of anaphylactic reactions [16].

2.3 L-Asparaginase side effects

L-Aspa-induced adverse effects may be minor or severe and fatal. Some common adverse effects are related to the L-glutaminase coactivity including a decrease in the production of various essential proteins such as albumin, insulin, fibrinogen, and protein-C [17]. So, L-Aspa may induce fever, hepatic dysfunction, hyperglycemia and diabetes, leucopenia, pancreatitis, neurological convulsions, and coagulation abnormalities such as thrombosis and hemorrhage [17].

Hypersensitivity life-threatening reactions may occur on asparaginase-based medications, causing edema, skin eruption, serum sickness, bronchospasm, urticaria, and anaphylactic shock [17].

3. Asparaginase-associated pancreatitis (AAP)

3.1 Definition

AAP is defined as acute pancreatitis occurring in patients receiving L-Aspa treatment at the time of onset of symptoms [18]. Pancreatitis is defined as the histological presence of inflammation within the pancreatic parenchyma. Acute pancreatitis is a reversible process characterized by the presence of interstitial edema, infiltration by acute inflammatory cells, and varying degrees of apoptosis, necrosis, and hemorrhage [19].

In various clinical trials, pancreatitis has been reported in 2–18% of patients undergoing L-Aspa therapy for ALL, with grade 3/4 pancreatitis occurring in 5–10% of patients [20, 21].

3.2 Pathophysiology

The exact pathogenesis of AAP is still unclear, but it may be related to the reduction in protein synthesis resulting from asparaginase-induced depletion of asparagine [18, 21].

Moreover, genetic predispositions are likely to play an important role. AAP occurs even after one or a few administrations of the drug with a high likelihood of recurrence upon re-exposure [21].

3.3 Diagnosis

Diagnosis of pancreatitis is based on a combination of clinical, biological (amylase, lipase), and radiological evidence.

3.3.1 Clinical presentation

In children, abdominal pain has many characteristics but is still the most common symptom of acute pancreatitis, occurring in 87% of cases. Abdominal pain in acute pancreatitis is of acute onset, especially in the epigastric region accompanied by nausea and vomiting [22].

3.3.2 Biochemical markers

Generally, amylasemia and lipasemia exceeding three times the upper normal level confirm the diagnosis. In pediatric patients, the simultaneous elevation of both pancreatic enzymes increases the sensitivity of the test to 94%. Thus, the analysis of both enzymes is recommended, especially in very young children [23].

3.3.3 Imaging methods

Imaging methods in AAP are based on ultrasonography and computerized tomography (CT). The main sonographic signs are increased pancreatic size and decreased pancreatic echogenicity. While, in mild cases, a normal gland can be observed, increased pancreatic size and decreased echogenicity may be reported in severe cases [24, 25]. When performed days or weeks after the onset of AAP, contrast-enhanced CT is used to identify pancreatic necrosis. Concerning the usage of magnetic resonance imaging (MRI), there are currently no recommendations.

Adult studies demonstrate that MRI provides roughly the same information as CT, although the evidence in children is limited [26].

3.3.4 Diagnostic criteria

In a child presenting with abdominal pain during cancer treatment, acute pancreatitis should always be considered and ruled out. The diagnosis of AP requires at least 2 of 3 criteria according to the INSPPIRE Project (International Study Group of Pediatric Pancreatitis: In Search for a Cure) [27]:

a. Abdominal pain caused by AP is frequently of sudden onset, especially in the epigastric region, and may radiate to the shoulder, accompanied by nausea or vomiting.

b. Serum amylase and/or lipase activity at least three times higher than normal (in international units/liter).

c. Imaging findings suggestive of AP (e.g., transabdominal ultrasonography, contrast-enhanced computerized tomography).

4. Early assessment of severity of APP

AAP is usually mild, not life-threatening, and responds favorably to intensive medical treatment. Several scores have been developed to assess the severity of AP. (For example, Ranson, Balthazar, SOFA, APACHE II, and Marshall scores). Outside of clinical trials, none of these indicators are commonly used in clinical practice [28].

The Harmless Acute Pancreatitis Score (HAPS) is a German-developed score that may reliably identify mild types of pancreatitis at the time of admission [29].

This score was created by combining three parameters that best predicted a non-severe course (no signs of peritonitis (rebound tenderness, guarding), normal hematocrit level, and normal serum creatinine level ≤ 2 mg/dl).

To identify patients at high risk of severe pancreatitis, the Bedside Index for Severity in Acute Pancreatitis (BISAP) score can be used [30]. This score has five parameters:

B unconjugated Bilirubin level > 25 mg/dl.
I Impaired mental status (Glasgow Coma Scale score < 15).

DOI: http://dx.doi.org/10.5772/intechopen.110034

S Development of systemic inflammatory response syndrome (SIRS).
A Age > 60 years.
P Presence of pleural effusion.

With an 83% sensitivity, a BISAP score of three or above can indicate a severe course of AP.

The Pancreatitis Activity Scoring System (PASS) recently expanded its severity criteria to include organ failure, pain, intolerance to a solid diet, systemic inflammatory response syndrome, and morphine equivalent dosage by relative weight [31].

However, these grading methods have not been verified in the pediatric population. On admission, different clinical and laboratory criteria may suggest moderate or severe AP, although variable threshold levels frequently complicate matters. However, in children, a high C-reactive protein (>150 mg/l), hypocalcemia, an elevated hematocrit, or hyperglycemia are more likely to suggest a severe course of pancreatitis [32].

According to the 2012 Atlanta criteria, pancreatitis is classified as mild, moderate, or severe [33]. Mild acute pancreatitis was defined by the absence of organ failure and local complications. Moderately severe acute pancreatitis was defined by local complications and/or transitory organ failure (<48 h) and severe acute pancreatitis was defined by persistent organ failure >48 h. Organ failure often includes respiratory, renal, or cardiovascular failure, requiring admission to an intermediate or intensive care unit. The revised Atlanta criteria are widely used by pediatricians in the classification of pancreatitis severity although not validated in this population. Until a consensus on the classification of AAP is reached among pediatric oncologists, we recommend that the Atlanta criteria are applied. L-Asparaginase is among the most trigger causes of severe acute pancreatitis [34].

5. Risk factors for AAP

5.1 Genetic predisposition

Genetic predisposition is suggested to play an important role in the occurrence of AAP. Although nucleotide sequence variants in several genes (e.g., CFTR, CTRC, PRSS1, and PRSS2) have been associated with the risk of pancreatitis in general [35], no specific genetic polymorphisms have been associated with AAP.

In 2016, Liu et al. identified a nonsense variant of the CPA2 gene, which encodes carboxypeptidase A2, associated with a higher predisposition risk of AAP [36].

5.2 Age

Higher age is associated with a higher risk of AAP. When compared to younger children, children above the age of 10 at the time of diagnosis had an increased risk of developing AAP [37].

5.3 Severe hypertriglyceridemia

In the presence of severe hypertriglyceridemia (i.e., levels above 11.3 mmol/l), the risk of acute pancreatitis is increased even in patients not receiving L-Aspa [38].

Hypertriglyceridemia is frequently observed in patients treated with L-Aspa, especially when given in combination with steroids [39].

5.4 Formulations of L-asparaginase

Alvarez and Zimmerman investigated the prevalence of pancreatitis in patients given different formulations of L-Aspa: PEG-asparaginase versus L-Aspa. The authors reported that the PEG asparaginase group had a statistically significant increase in pancreatitis when compared to the control group. (18% PEG-asparaginase vs. 1.9% L-Aspa, $p = 0.007$) [40]. This effect was explained by a longer half-life of PEG-asparaginase resulting in prolonged asparagine depletion.

In contrast, other studies have found no difference in pancreatitis frequency between PEG-asparaginase and L-Aspa patients [41, 42].

5.5 ALL risk stratification and L-Aspa dosing

In two studies, patients in the high-risk ALL stratification group had a higher incidence of AAP, receiving the highest doses of asparaginase [21, 43]. In Raja and colleagues' study, the high-risk stratification group received lower doses of asparaginase and had a lower rate of AAP [20]. These findings suggest that a higher cumulative dose of asparaginase may be associated with a higher incidence of AAP.

6. Treatment

Actually, there is no pharmacological treatment for acute pancreatitis whether it is primary or secondary. The therapeutic approach of AAP is identical to that of the pancreatitis of other etiologies. Treatment of AAP is primarily supportive and aims to reduce symptoms and monitor potential complications after immediate discontinuation of L-Aspa [21, 40, 44].

Patients with acute pancreatitis should be clinically examined for symptoms of organ failure to be appropriately treated immediately.

6.1 Fluid resuscitation

Circulatory anomalies are frequent in patients with severe sepsis or septic shock and must be managed in an intensive care unit. Early administration of adequate fluid resuscitation to avoid hypovolemia and organ hypoperfusion is a major pillar of management [45].

Numerous studies have investigated the type and amount of intravenous fluid resuscitation in severe AP. Keystones in fluid resuscitation are the followings:

a. Appropriate intravenous fluid resuscitation should be done within the first 24–48 hours; postponed or deficient fluids decrease the survival rate [45, 46].

b. High-volume fluid treatment (1000 mL/h) may increase the mortality rate and should be prevented [47].

c. Ringer's lactate is the optimum fluid to use. During the first 24 hours, the infusion rate should be assessed on a frequent basis and adjusted based on urine excretion (target: 0.5–1 mL/kg/h) and vital parameters. The recommended infusion rate is 250–500 ml/h unless there are cardiovascular, renal, or other related comorbidities [48, 49].

Goal-directed therapy typically focuses on heart rate, mean arterial pressure, central venous pressure, urine output, blood urea nitrogen concentration, and hematocrit [2].

6.2 Analgesia

Opioid (e.g., pethidine) and non-opioid (e.g., metamizole) analgesics are indicated. In fact, pain is a distress condition that must be managed with adequate intravenous analgesia. If intravenous analgesia fails to provide sufficient relief or enhances bowel paralysis, the use of thoracic epidural analgesia may be considered. This pain-relieving technique was associated with improved survival in a multicenter retrospective trial [50]. A recent study showed a beneficial trend but no significant improvement in organ dysfunction or mortality upon thoracic epidural analgesia [51].

6.3 Enteral feeding

Based on several randomized clinical trials of non-asparaginase-related pancreatitis in adults, early enteral feeding seems to reduce the incidence of complications [44, 52]. Nutrition most likely protects the mucosal barrier and reduces bacterial translocation in the gut, decreasing the risk of infection and necrosis [52]. This is contrary to earlier beliefs. However, studies on children are lacking.

6.4 Prophylactic antibiotics/protease inhibitors

There is no clear evidence of the benefits of routine use of antibiotics in the early course of severe acute pancreatitis [53]. A recent study including more than 800 patients showed that antibiotic prophylaxis in patients with severe AP may lead to the development of invasive candidiasis of the pancreas [54]. Further studies must clarify the benefice of antimicrobial prophylaxis in certain subgroups of severe AP. Intravenous antibiotics are recommended in the case of cholangitis or other local infections, for example, infected walled-off necrosis.

More rarely applied treatments in case of severe pancreatitis are the administration of the synthetic somatostatin analog Octreotide or continuous regional arterial infusion of protease inhibitors and antibiotics [55, 56]. In fact, Somatostatin (Octreotide) inhibits secretions of the pancreatic digestive enzymes leading to a decrease in pancreatic inflammation [55].

There are no large studies of Octreotide treatment in children with AAP or other children with AP. In addition, there is no consensus on doses, duration, and the pattern of side effects. In the case reports, patients were treated with doses that ranged from 2.5 to 7.2 μg/kg per day [56].

Continuous regional arterial infusion of protease inhibitors and antibiotics are shown to be effective in preventing complications and in reducing mortality rates in severe acute pancreatitis in a large adult trial [57].

Pediatric data is still insufficient. Five pediatric patients with severe AAP were treated with continuous regional arterial infusion within 48 hours of diagnosis in one trial [58]. After 22 days, all five patients had satisfactory clinical results and could continue chemotherapy, despite the fact that none received further L-Aspa treatment [58].

7. Complications of AAP

Acute severe complications following AP include systemic inflammatory response syndrome and multiorgan failure affecting most frequently lungs and kidneys. Patients may develop pleural effusions, toxic pneumonia, acute respiratory distress syndrome, and renal failure [59].

7.1 Short-term complications

Short-term complications, usually appearing after the first week, include the development of life-threatening systemic inflammatory response syndrome and multiorgan failure. Other complications include necrosis and infection [18].

Pseudocysts can emerge as a complication to AAP. Such cysts contain pancreatic juice enclosed by a non-epithelialized wall [60]. Although most pseudocysts have been observed to arise within 4 weeks after acute pancreatitis [60], there are no significant studies that document this in detail for AAP patients. In general, pseudocysts should be treated conservatively, as the majority of instances diminish after a few weeks or months [22].

Intervention is indicated in patients that have persistent symptoms, such as severe pain, despite supportive care, or in case of infection or bleeding [61].

7.2 Long-term complications

Long-term consequences include diabetes mellitus, persistent abdominal discomfort, and chronic pancreatitis [15, 21, 22, 40]. It was demonstrated that the risk of the enduring requirement for insulin medication and recurring abdominal pain was related to having had pseudocysts [14].

8. Re-introduction of L-asparaginase

In children with ALL, suspending asparaginase therapy after toxicity is associated with significantly decreased event-free survival [4]. It is, therefore, crucial that ALL protocols include recommendations regarding the re-introduction of L-Aspa treatment after AAP.

Five studies have described the re-administration of L-Aspa after the occurrence of AAP [20, 43, 60–63]. The rate of AAP when L-Aspa was re-introduced was reported to be 0% (0 out of one patient) [62], 7, 7% (two out of 26 patients) [63], 25% (1 out of 4 patients) [43], 63% (10 out 16 patients) [64] and 17% (2 out 12 patients) [20]. The difference in the incidence of AAP after reintroduction of L-Aspa in the two larger studies primarily reflects the criteria for reintroduction, being mild AAP and complete resolution of symptoms in one study [63], whereas the other study only required resolution of symptoms within 72 h [64].

Currently, there are no established guidelines for the reintroduction of asparaginase following an episode of pancreatitis.

Based on the current literature and the Atlanta criteria, Raja et al. [18] suggested that in cases where patients with AAP had a rapid resolution of clinical symptoms and a reduction in serum amylase and lipase to levels less than three times the upper limit of normal within 48 hours of being diagnosed with pancreatitis and did not have signs of severity such as a pancreatic pseudocyst or necrosis, reintroduction of L-Aspa

DOI: http://dx.doi.org/10.5772/intechopen.110034

could be attempted. If a second episode of pancreatitis occurs after reintroducing L-Aspa, asparaginase medication should be avoided completely. These findings suggest that clinicians should be conscious of the relatively high risk of recurrent pancreatitis with asparaginase reexposure following a first episode of AAP.

9. Conclusion

AAP is a life-threatening complication of ALL therapy and there is a need for consensus on its definition in all L-Aspa-containing protocols. Monitoring the patients treated with L-Aspa, through careful observation of clinical signs and laboratory follow-up is crucial to early detect asparaginase-associated toxicity to enable effective and appropriate management and recognize cases where re-exposure is possible.

Conflict of interest

The authors declare no conflict of interest.

Notes/thanks/other declarations

Thanks to all authors who contributed to this work.

Abbreviations

L-Aspa	L-Asparaginase
ALL	Acute lymphoblastic leukemia
AP	Acute pancreatitis
AAP	Asparaginase-associated pancreatitis
ASNS	Asparagine synthetase
CT	Computerized tomography
MRI	Magnetic resonance imaging
HAPS	The harmless acute pancreatitis score
BISAP	The bedside index for severity in acute pancreatitis
PASS	The pancreatitis activity scoring system

Author details

Kmira Zahra[1*], Wided Cherif[1], Naila Fathallah[2], Haifa Regaieg[1], Monia Zaier[1], Yosra Ben Youssef[1] and Abderrahim Khelif[1]

1 Department of Clinical Hematology, Farhat Hached Hospital, Sousse, Tunisia

2 Department of Pharmacology, Farhat Hached Hospital, Sousse, Tunisia

*Address all correspondence to: kmira_zahra@yahoo.fr

References

[1] Hijiya N, van der Sluis IM. Asparaginase-associated toxicity in children with acute lymphoblastic leukemia. Leukemia & Lymphoma. 2015;**8194**:1-31

[2] Müller HJ, Boos J. Use of L-asparaginase in childhood ALL. Critical Reviews in Oncology/ Hematology. 1998;**28**:97-113

[3] Pession A, Valsecchi MG, Masera G, et al. Long-term results of a randomized trial on extended use of high dose L-asparaginase for standard risk childhood acute lymphoblastic leukemia. Journal of Clinical Oncology. 2005;**23**:7161-7167

[4] Silverman LB. Improved outcome for children with acute lymphoblastic leukemia: Results of Dana-Farber Consortium Protocol 91-01. Blood. 2001;**97**:1211-1218

[5] Asselin BL, Whitin JC, Coppola DJ, Rupp IP, Sallan SE, Cohen HJ. Comparative pharmacokinetic studies of three asparaginase preparations. Journal of Clinical Oncology. 1993;**11**:1780-1786

[6] Pinkel D. Treatment of childhood acute lymphocytic leukemia. The Journal of Pediatrics. 1970;**77**:1089-1091

[7] Van Trimpont M, Schalk AM, De Visser Y, Nguyen HA, Reunes L, Vandemeulebroecke K, et al. In vivo stabilization of a less toxic asparaginase variant leads to a durable anti-tumor response in acute leukemia. Haematologica. 2022;**2022**:18

[8] Boos J, Werber G, Ahlke E, et al. Monitoring of asparaginase activity and asparagine levels in children on different asparaginase preparations. European Journal of Cancer. 1996;**32A**:1544-1550

[9] Appel IM, Kazemier KM, Boos J, et al. Pharmacokinetic, pharmacodynamic and intracellular effects of PEG-asparaginase in newly diagnosed childhood acute lymphoblastic leukemia: Results from a single agent window study. Leukemia. 2008;**22**:1665-1679

[10] Panetta JC, Gajjar A, Hijiya N, et al. Comparison of native E. coli and PEG asparaginase pharmacokinetics and pharmacodynamics in pediatric acute lymphoblastic leukemia. Clinical Pharmacology and Therapeutics. 2009;**86**:651-658

[11] Duval M, Suciu S, Ferster A, Rialland X, Nelken B, Lutz P, et al. Comparison of Escherichia coli-asparaginase with Erwinia-asparaginase in the treatment of childhood lymphoid malignancies: Results of a randomized European Organisation for Research and Treatment of Cancer-Children's Leukemia Group phase 3 trial. Blood. 2002;**99**:2734-2739

[12] Covini D, Tardito S, Bussolati O, et al. Expanding targets for a metabolic therapy of cancer: L-asparaginase. Recent Patents on Anti-Cancer Drug Discovery. 2012;**7**:4-13

[13] Moola ZB, Scawen MD, Atkinson T, et al. Erwinia chrysanthemi L-asparaginase: Epitope mapping and production of antigenically modified enzymes. The Biochemical Journal. 1994;**302**:921-927

[14] Salzer W, Seibel N, Smith M. Erwinia asparaginase in pediatric acute lymphoblastic leukemia. Expert Opinion on Biological Therapy. 2012;**12**:1407-1414

[15] Wolthers BO, Frandsen TL, Baruchel A, Attarbaschi A, Barzilai S, Colombini A, et al. Asparaginase-associated pancreatitis in childhood acute lymphoblastic leukaemia: An observational Ponte di Legno Toxicity Working Group study. Lancet Oncology. 2017;**18**(9):1238-1248

[16] Spiegel RJ, Echelberger CK, Poplack DG. Delayed allergic reactions following intramuscular L-asparaginase. Medical and Pediatric Oncology. 1980;**8**(2):123-125

[17] Fonseca MHG, da Fiúza T, de Morais SB, de Souza T, de Trevizani R. Circumventing the side effects of L-asparaginase. Biomedicine & Pharmacotherapy. 2021;**139**:111616

[18] Raja RA, Schmiegelow K, Frandsen TL. Asparaginase-associated pancreatitis in children. British Journal of Haematology. 2012;**159**(1):18-27

[19] Bradley EL III. A clinically based classification system for acute pancreatitis. Summary of the International Symposium on Acute Pancreatitis, Atlanta, Ga, September 11 through 13, 1992. Archives of Surgery. 1993;**128**:586-590

[20] Raja RA, Schmiegelow K, Albertsen BK, et al. Asparaginase-associated pancreatitis in children with acute lymphoblastic leukaemia in the NOPHO ALL2008 protocol. British Journal of Haematology. 2014;**165**:126-133

[21] Treepongkaruna S, Thongpak N, Pakakasama S, Pienvichit P, Sirachainan N, Hongeng S. Acute pancreatitis in children with acute lymphoblastic leukemia after chemotherapy. Journal of Pediatric Hematology/Oncology. 2009;**31**(11):812-815

[22] Bai HX, Lowe ME, Husain SZ. What have we learned about acute pancreatitis in children? Journal of Pediatric Gastroenterology and Nutrition. 2011;**52**:262-270

[23] Yadav D, Agarwal N, Pitchumoni CS. A critical evaluation of laboratory tests in acute pancreatitis. The American Journal of Gastroenterology. 2002;**97**:1309-1318

[24] Mader TJ, McHugh TP. Acute pancreatitis in children. Pediatric Emergency Care. 1992;**8**:157-161

[25] Elmas N. The role of diagnostic radiology in pancreatitis. European Journal of Radiology. 2001;**38**:120-132

[26] Tipnis NA, Dua KS, Werlin SL. A retrospective assessment of magnetic resonance cholangiopancreatography in children. Journal of Pediatric Gastroenterology and Nutrition. 2002;**46**:59-64

[27] Morinville VD, Husain SZ, Bai H, Barth B, Alhosh R, Dure PR, et al. Definitions of pediatric pancreatitis and survey of present clinical practices. Journal of Pediatric Gastroenterology and Nutrition. 2012;**55**:261-265

[28] Gliem N, Ammer-Herrmenau C, Ellenrieder V, Neesse A. Management of severe acute pancreatitis: An update. Digestion. 2021;**102**(4):503-507

[29] Lankisch PG, Weber-Dany B, Hebel K, Maisonneuve P, Lowenfels AB. The harmless acute pancreatitis score: A clinical algorithm for rapid initial stratification of nonsevere disease. Clinical Gastroenterology Hepatology. 2009;**7**(6):702-705

[30] Singh VK, Wu BU, Bollen TL, Repas K, Maurer R, Johannes RS, et al. A prospective evaluation of the bedside index for severity in acute pancreatitis

score in assessing mortality and intermediate markers of severity in acute pancreatitis. American Journal of Gastroenterology. 2009;**104**(4):966-971

[31] Buxbaum J, Quezada M, Chong B, Gupta N, Yu CY, Lane C, et al. The pancreatitis activity scoring system predicts clinical outcomes in acute pancreatitis: Findings from a prospective cohort study. American Journal of Gastroenterology. 2018;**113**(5):755-764

[32] Brown A, Baillargeon JD, Hughes MD, Banks PA. Can fluid resuscitation prevent pancreatic necrosis in severe acute pancreatitis? Pancreatology. 2002;**2**(2):104-107

[33] Banks PA, Bollen TL, Dervenis C, Gooszen HG, Johnson CD, Sarr MG, et al. Classification of acute pancreatitis—2012: Revision of the Atlanta classification and definitions by international consensus. Gut. 2013;**62**(1):102-111

[34] Szabo FK, Hornung L, Oparaji JA, Alhosh R, Husain SZ, Liu QY, et al. A prognostic tool to predict severe acute pancreatitis in pediatrics. Pancreatology. 2016;**16**(3):358-364

[35] Whitcomb DC. Genetic aspects of pancreatitis. Annual Review of Medicine. 2010;**61**:413-424

[36] Liu C, Yang W, Devidas M, Cheng C, Pei D, Smith C, et al. Clinical and genetic risk factors for acute pancreatitis in patients with acute lymphoblastic leukemia. Journal of Clinical Oncology. 2016;**34**(18):2133-2140

[37] Oparaji JA, Rose F, Okafor D, Howard A, Turner RL, Orabi AI, et al. Risk factors for Asparaginase-associated pancreatitis: A systematic review. Journal of Clinical Gastroenterology. 2017;**51**(10):907-913

[38] Yadav D, Pitchumoni CS. Issues in hyperlipidemic pancreatitis. Journal of Clinical Gastroenterology. 2003;**36**:54-62

[39] Parsons SK, Skapek SX, Neufeld EJ, Kuhlman C, Young ML, Donnelly M, et al. Asparaginase- associated lipid abnormalities in children with acute lymphoblastic leukemia. Blood. 1997;**89**:1886-1895

[40] Alvarez OA, Zimmerman G. Pegaspargase-induced pancreatitis. Medicine Pediatric Oncology. 2000;**34**(3):200-205

[41] Kurtzberg J, Asselin B, Bernstein M, Buchanan GR, Pollock BH, Camitta BM. Polyethylene glycol-conjugated L-asparaginase versus native L-asparaginase in combination with standard agents for children with acute lymphoblastic leukemia in second bone marrow relapse: A Children's Oncology Group Study (POG 8866). Journal of Pediatric Hematology Oncology. 2011;**33**(8):610-616

[42] Place AE, Stevenson KE, Vrooman LM, Harris MH, Hunt SK, O'Brien JE, et al. Intravenous pegylated asparaginase versus intramuscular native Escherichia coli L-asparaginase in newly diagnosed childhood acute lymphoblastic leukaemia (DFCI 05-001): A randomised, open-label phase 3 trial. Lancet Oncology. 2015;**16**(16):1677-1690

[43] Samarasinghe S, Dhir S, Slack J, Iyer P, Wade R, Clack R, et al. Incidence and outcome of pancreatitis in children and young adults with acute lymphoblastic leukaemia treated on a contemporary protocol, UKALL 2003. British Journal of Haematology. 2013;**162**(5):710-713

[44] Wu XM, Ji KQ, Wang HY, Li GF, Zang B, Chen WM. Total enteral nutrition in prevention of pancreatic

necrotic infection in severe acute pancreatitis. Pancreas. 2010;**39**:248-251

[45] Gardner TB, Vege SS, Chari ST, Petersen BT, Topazian MD, Clain JE, et al. Faster rate of initial fluid resuscitation in severe acute pancreatitis diminishes in-hospital mortality. Pancreatology. 2009;**9**:770-776

[46] Warndorf MG, Kurtzman JT, Bartel MJ, Cox M, Mackenzie T, Robinson S, et al. Early fluid resuscitation reduces morbidity among patients with acute pancreatitis. Clinical Gastroenterology and Hepatology. 2011;**9**(8):705-709

[47] Mao EQ, Fei J, Peng YB, Huang J, Tang YQ, Zhang SD. Rapid hemodilution is associated with increased sepsis and mortality among patients with severe acute pancreatitis. Chinese Medical Journal. 2010;**123**(13):1639-1644

[48] James TW, Crockett SD. Management of acute pancreatitis in the first 72 hours. Current Opinion in Gastroenterology. 2018;**34**(5):330-335

[49] Tenner S, Baillie J, Dewitt J, Vege SS, American College of Gastroenterology. American College of Gastroenterology guideline: Management of acute pancreatitis. American Journal of Gastroenterology. 2013;**108**(9):1400-1415

[50] Jabaudon M, Belhadj-Tahar N, Rimmelé T, Joannes-Boyau O, Bulyez S, Lefrant JY, et al. Thoracic epidural analgesia and mortality in acute pancreatitis: A Multicenter propensity analysis. Critical Care Medicine. 2018;**46**(3):e198-e205

[51] Tyagi A, Gupta YR, Das S, Rai G, Gupta A. Effect of segmental thoracic epidural block on pancreatitis induced organ dysfunction: A preliminary study. Indian Journal of Critical Care Medicine. 2019;**23**(2):89-84

[52] Petrov MS, Kukosh MV, Emelyanov NV. A randomized controlled trial of enteral versus parenteral feeding in patients with predicted severe acute pancreatitis shows a significant reduction in mortality and in infected pancreatic complications with total enteral nutrition. Digestive Surgery. 2006;**23**:336-344

[53] Arlt A, Erhart W, Schafmayer C, Held HC, Hampe J. Antibiosis of necrotizing pancreatitis. Viszeralmedizin. 2014;**30**(5):318-324

[54] Horibe M, Sanui M, Sasaki M, Honda H, Ogura Y, Namiki S. et al, Impact of antimicrobial prophylaxis for severe acute pancreatitis on the development of invasive candidiasis: a large retrospective multicenter cohort study. Pancreas. 2019;**48**(4):537-543

[55] Takeda K, Matsuno S, Ogawa M, Watanabe S, Atomi Y. Continuous regional arterial infusion (CRAI) therapy reduces the mortality rate of acute necrotizing pancreatitis: Results of a cooperative survey in Japan. Journal of Hepato- Biliary-Pancreatic Surgery. 2001;**8**:216-220

[56] Garrington T, Bensard D, Ingram JD, Silliman CC. Successful management with octreotide of a child with L-asparaginase induced hemorrhagic pancreatitis. Medical and Pediatric Oncology. 1998;**30**:106-109

[57] Piascik M, Rydzewska G, Milewski J, Olszewski S, Furmanek M, Walecki J, et al. The results of severe acute pancreatitis treatment with continuous regional arterial infusion of protease inhibitor and antibiotic: A randomized controlled study. Pancreas. 2010;**39**:863-867

[58] Morimoto A, Imamura T, Ishii R, Nakabayashi Y, Nakatani T, Sakagami J,

et al. Successful management of severe L-asparaginase- associated pancreatitis by continuous regional arterial infusion of protease inhibitor and antibiotic. Cancer. 2008;**113**:1362-1369

[59] Pastor CM, Matthay MA, Frossard JL. Pancreatitis-associated acute lung injury: New insights. Chest. 2003;**124**:2341-2351

[60] Banks PA, Freeman ML. Practice guidelines in acute pancreatitis. The American Journal of Gastroenterology. 2006;**101**:2379-2400

[61] Gumaste VV, Aron J. Pseudocyst management: Endoscopic drainage and other emerging techniques. Journal of Clinical Gastroenterology. 2010;**44**:326-331

[62] Vrooman LM, Supko JG, Neuberg DS, Asselin BL, Athale UH, Clavell L, et al. Erwinia asparaginase after allergy to E. coli asparaginase in children with acute lymphoblastic leukemia. Pediatric Blood and Cancer. 2010;**54**:199-205

[63] Knoderer HM, Robarge J, Flockhart DA. Predicting asparaginase-associated pancreatitis. Pediatric Blood and Cancer. 2007;**49**:634-639

[64] Kearney SL, Dahlberg SE, Levy DE, et al. Clinical course and outcome in children with acute lymphoblastic leukemia and asparaginase-associated pancreatitis. Pediatric Blood & Cancer. 2009;**53**:162-167